Stepping Forward

A Runner's Guide to Moving for Life

"Eat well and run and/or walk for the rest of your life."

Howard Elakman

RRCA & USATF Certified Running Coach

iUniverse, Inc.
New York Bloomington

Stepping Forward
A Runner's Guide to Moving for Life

Copyright © 2009 by Howard Elakman.

All rights reserved. No part of this book may be used or reproduced by any means, graphic, electronic, or mechanical, including photocopying, recording, taping or by any information storage retrieval system without the written permission of the publisher except in the case of brief quotations embodied in critical articles and reviews.

The information, ideas, and suggestions in this book are not intended as a substitute for professional medical advice. Before following any suggestions contained in this book, you should consult your personal physician. Neither the author nor the publisher shall be liable or responsible for any loss or damage allegedly arising as a consequence of your use or application of any information or suggestions in this book.

iUniverse books may be ordered through booksellers or by contacting:

iUniverse
1663 Liberty Drive
Bloomington, IN 47403
www.iuniverse.com
1-800-Authors (1-800-288-4677)

Because of the dynamic nature of the Internet, any Web addresses or links contained in this book may have changed since publication and may no longer be valid. The views expressed in this work are solely those of the author and do not necessarily reflect the views of the publisher, and the publisher hereby disclaims any responsibility for them.

ISBN: 978-0-595-50778-8 (pbk)
ISBN: 978-0-595-63576-4 (cloth)
ISBN: 978-0-595-61644-2 (ebk)

Printed in the United States of America

iUniverse rev. date: 5/8/2009

Contents

Acknowledgments vii
Introduction xiii

Part 1   **Warming Up** 1
One   Before Beginning .3
Two   Getting Started 11
Three   Preparing Mentally 27

Part 2   **Taking Off** 33
Four   Training 35
Five   Stretching & Muscle Enhancement 47
Six   Nutrition 71
Seven   Safety Precautions 77

Appendix A   Down the Road 81
Appendix B   Marathons: What to Expect 83
Appendix C   A Marathon Timeline 89
Appendix D   Injury Free Running 93
Appendix E   Schedules for Marathon and Half Marathon . .95

             References 111

Acknowledgments

I would like to thank my wife, Rosanne, for her assistance and patience with me during the writing of this book.

I also want to thank Dr. Janet E. Parke for her suggestions, editing, and support with the writing of this book. I am not sure I could have even started writing without her help.

The artwork for all the stretches and strength improvements was done by my granddaughter, Abigail Elakman. She is fourteen years old and a great artist, but save these drawings and eventually they will be collectors' items. Thank you, Abigail!

FOREWORD

Did you ever think that running around in circles would get you places?

The purpose of circling the track, at various speeds for various distances, under the supervision of a trained coach with a critical eye, enables him to evaluate your correct posture, pace, and stride. These are the basic elements of running.

The sport of running can be a lifelong enjoyment, if practiced in a healthy disciplined manner. Keeping fit by running is likened to the new fountain of youth. Research shows that vigorous exercise helps prevent heart attacks, aid in weight control, and instills a feeling of well-being while enhancing creativity as well. Medically it has been found to help patients with diabetes, ulcers, nervous tension, high blood pressure, back pain, as well as depression, recurring headaches, and menstrual cramps. It benefits the symptoms of hangovers, jet lag, constipation, and insomnia.

Keeping a fit body may accomplish all of the above, but preventing running injuries and stress, due to overuse syndromes, must be foremost. With the guidance of this book as your first step, you will minimize any possibility of trauma to the body. Problems incurred by running improperly may be understood when the following comparison between walking and running is explained.

An average 150 lb. man walking with a normal step length of 2.5 ft. will absorb 80% of his body weight at ground contact, or 127 tons per mile. Conversely, running for the same mile and taking a step of 3.5 ft. will absorb 250% of body weight at ground contact, or 220 tons per mile. Therefore, any weakness, faulty biomechanics, or improper running technique shall be exaggerated due to the impact of doubling of the gravitational forces.

I have personally run with the author, Howard Elakman, for over 25 years. I have personally completed five marathons and hundreds of shorter races. I am well aware of the complexity of running properly and injury free. During this period of time, Howard Elakman has demonstrated knowledge and skill by correcting many of my prior faulty habits. His advice has been sought by many regional runners who have successfully completed marathons who previously thought this was unachievable.

As a podiatrist specializing in orthopedics and surgery, I have admired and recognized his coaching acumen.

Studying this guide will enable you to run safely and comfortably for many healthy years. Enjoy learning and running.

Dr. Harvey J. Saff
Diplomate, American Board of Podiatric Orthopedics
Diplomate, American Board of Podiatric Surgery
Fellow, American College of Podiatric Sports Medicine

Introduction

How does one start running or walking? I went out for track in high school, but our coach believed that if you did not throw up during or after practice you were not putting out 100 percent. This turned me off completely, and I looked for other activities. I played golf because it was a good way to get in a five-mile walk. Then golf carts arrived on the scene, and it suddenly seemed foolish to ride around so I could swing my arms over a hundred times. I gave that up and started playing four-wall handball. This was a great game which forced me to use both hands. After a few years it became impossible to find a game because everyone was playing racket ball. There went the use of my left hand.

When I was at the age of thirty-eight, a friend convinced me to run with him. I really didn't like the idea of it, but there wasn't anything else that interested me and I was gaining weight. Since I love to eat, I stayed with running. I have not been sorry, because I came into a whole new world. I met some of the most wonderful people, joined groups of runners, and went to races all over the world. In 2002, I gained certification with the Road Runner's Club of America (RRCA) and still take continuing education courses with them. In 2003, I received my level-one certification from USA Track and Field (USATF). And I still love to eat.

Now that I am getting older and walk more than I run, I have to start watching how much I eat. The great thing about running is that when you are running fifty to seventy-five miles every week, you can eat a lot and not gain weight. You can even cheat and have dessert. I try not to let running be my whole life. However, I am very active in the running community and think it is a great life. I, and my wife, have friends to walk and run with and can maintain a healthy way of life.

Hopefully this book will help you find a similar experience. *Stepping Forward* is not intended for anyone who can run a 5K at a seven-minute pace or better. This book is intended for new runners and walkers. If you want to run or walk a marathon, half marathon, or any shorter-distance race and are interested in learning how or want to improve, then read on. In this book, you will learn how to run and/or walk, the clothing required, what to eat, what to drink, stretching to improve flexibility, other exercises for good body condition, and the mental attitude necessary to continue to maintain a healthy body and lifestyle.

Today is the first day of the rest of your life, so make the best of it. Start thinking about running and/or walking for the rest of your life. Make the decision to step forward, live healthy, and be happy.

Part One

Warming Up

Chapter One
Before Beginning

The new runner can be one that is overweight and has been thinking about getting started, but something else always takes priority. Establishing a priority for a new healthy way of life should take precedence. Some think that they can't run a block, but after a month with me they find that they actually can run.

I generally place runners in three different categories:

1) The natural runner who runs with no lessons and does everything right. He is competitive and looks to beat anyone in front of him.

2) The runner who takes the time to get proper instruction from someone who has studied and learned what is required to run with the best form and what is required for stretching, strengthening, eating correctly, and mentally approaching the task of competition.

3) Finally, everyone else who believes that putting one foot in front of the other is all there is to it. There is

nothing wrong with this if that is all you want from your exercise program.

Based on the descriptions above, you should be able to place yourself within one of those three categories. Regardless of which category you fall under, as long as you are putting out the effort, why not get the most out of it? Even if you run fairly fast, you can run even faster and avoid injury at the same time.

If you have been thinking of starting a running or walking program, I am sure that you have heard that running is bad for your knees. This is true if your knees are weak to begin with. I believe that you can run without injury if you strengthen your legs before or while you are learning to run. There is more to running than just putting one foot in front of the other. You must learn the correct form and you must strengthen your body from the waist to the bottom of your feet.

Running and Walking

But should you be running at all? To begin, let's take a look at the difference between running and walking. When running, you are airborne (high impact), and when walking, you always have one foot on the surface (low impact). If for some reason you cannot take the higher impact of running, you should stick to walking. You should not be a stroller, however. To get the benefit of walking as an exercise you must raise your heart rate by walking faster.

Race walkers can walk at an eight-minute-per-mile pace. You should be able to walk at a fifteen-minute pace or faster to gain the maximum benefit. As a stroller, you will find that the others will leave you. In most marathons, you will be picked up by the bus if you cannot reach a predetermined point by a certain time (check this before you register for the marathon or half marathon). Take your pick. There is no excuse for not being a runner, a walker, or a combination of both. You can run for a predetermined time and then walk for a predetermined time. Practice several different combinations to find what suits you best.

For example, the Galloway Method is to run for five minutes and walk for one minute and then repeat the cycle. You can start with a one-minute run and then walk for one minute and build slowly from there. What works best is up to the individual, though most healthy people will end up running because they want to join and stay with the crowd. Unfortunately, very overweight people tend to remain as walkers.

If you have not been exercising for a few years or if you are over forty-five years of age, it is advisable to check with your physician before starting a running or walking program. At the very least, go online and search for the PAR-Q form. This will bring you to the Physical Activity Readiness Questionnaire. Answer all of the questions to see how ready you are for exercise.

Remember that with any new sport you must learn to walk before you can run. The idea is to start slow and very gradually pick up the pace. Both pace and distance should be increased very gradually. Don't be embarrassed or ashamed if you can only run ten yards at a time when you start walking or running. The most important thing is to keep at it. A year later you will be impressed with yourself when you find that you can run a very long way without stopping. You will also be impressed with how you feel and how you look.

Join a club or a running group to find a partner who runs or walks at the same speed that you do. I can assure you that there is someone out there who is very similar to you, and you can support each other. Do an Internet search for RRCA, *Runner's World*, or running clubs in your area, or just visit a running store in your area. Any of these sources can get you connected with local runners. Enter a 5K race, even if you fear coming in last. You will not only gain experience, but you will surely meet someone who runs or walks just like you. It's a whole new world of running out there, and you will surely fit in.

Training Log

A training log is important so that you have a written account of your improvement. A sample entry could be 5 miles, 30:35 time, started at 6AM, drank V8 juice, temp. 55 degrees, circle around golf course, felt good. The date of course is on your log calendar. Any calendar will do, provided there is room to write short notes about what you did that day. If you can, comment on what you ate, how you felt, the weather, how far you went, whether you ran or walked, etc. Add anything you think you would like to know in the future about how you advanced.

Go to the *Runner's World* Web site on the Internet. In the past they have printed up small running log booklets. You can usually get one for free if you subscribe to the magazine. Local running stores also sell log books, but you do not need anything that formal. If you are computer savvy, you can set up an Excel program to keep track of your progress. Be sure to put enough columns in to cover date, time, the course, weather, what you ate before, after, and during exercise, and a larger column for any notes. It's always nice to look back and say, "That couldn't have been me," but more important, is to look back and see where you can improve.

Shoes

Shoes are really the only item that requires that you to do some shopping. Male or female, I will recommend that you go into a running store and try on every pair of shoes the store has in your size.

Walk around or even go out and run around the block. Find the pair that seems to fit you the best. Don't consider the color or how they look. Take the pair that feels the best. Wear them for two or three weeks, and if they still feel good, go back and buy another pair. You should always have two pairs so you can switch off every day and always have a dry pair of shoes.

The shoes do not have to be the top of the line. Running shoes will cost from sixty dollars on up to how much you want to pay or how much you can afford. The best investment is a good pair of running shoes that fit you properly. Good shoes will help you avoid getting injured. In your log you might consider keeping track of how many miles you have on the shoes that you are wearing. This could help you determine when you need new shoes.

If you plan on running a long time (two hours or more), bear in mind that your feet will expand. Get shoes that are at least a half size larger than your regular street shoes. Remember that running shoes are not bedroom slippers—they are there to help you run, to absorb the shock, and to become a part of your foot. Always lace them snugly so that they do not slip around while you are running. Laces should always be tied twice (double knot) so that they do not come apart when you are running. Having to stop during a race to tie your shoes is not a good idea.

A good running store can help you in the selection of your shoes. It is always a good idea to bring an old pair of running shoes with you when you want to buy new ones. The clerk will be able to tell from the wear if you are a pronator, meaning you put more weight on the inside of your feet, and what type of shoe would be best for you. Shoes designed for running will help to absorb the shock from the impact of running. When you get faster you might consider a pair of trainer shoes or racing flats for your track workouts (best on a rubberized track). After you have run two (2) or three (3) thousand miles, your feet and legs should be strong enough to do shorter races with a flat or trainer shoe.

Do not depend on shoes to do all the work. Your feet take the brunt of the force when running. Strengthening of the feet is an important thing to remember.

Clothing

What you wear should be comfortable and correct for the weather conditions. Some of the new fabrics that wick away perspiration work very well in warm weather. Several layers of clothing are better than one heavy garment for cold weather. You will warm up as you run, and you will probably want to remove one layer at a time.

Don't be a fashion model. During the longer races, you may have to throw away some clothes (it may get warm after a couple of hours, and you really don't want anything wrapped around you). Old and comfortable is better than new. At your marathon or half marathon, always be prepared for weather and bring a large garbage bag with a head hole cut out at the bottom. This comes in handy if you have to wait in the corral before a race starts. The bigger marathons (New York, Chicago, Marine Corps., etc.) have waiting areas set up where you group according to the time you have estimated for your finish (the pace you will run or walk at). These are the corrals. Each corral starts one after the other with the faster groups going first, and if you are in a slow-pace corral, you may be standing there for twenty, thirty, forty minutes, or more before you start. That plastic bag becomes an important item when you are in very cold temperatures. It can keep you warm and can be discarded just before you start.

During training you should have determined whether you like heavy socks or light weight socks. Which feel better on your feet? Decide on whether you need any of that greasy kid stuff on your feet (Crisco works well). There are several brands of lotion that can be rubbed into your feet before you put your socks on. By the time you are ready to run your race you should know how to avoid blisters. If you have done a good job strengthening your feet you probably won't need this.

To Review

- Decide whether you should start out running or walking. Have a plan based on your training.
- Check with your doctor before beginning any new exercise regimen.
- Keep a log so you can track your progress.
- Have at least two pair of proper shoes.
- Dress for the weather and not for the runway.

Chapter Two
Getting Started

You certainly should consider getting with a group or at least a partner to run or walk with. More than one person is desirable so that you can be sure to have a partner for every day that you run.

Remember that you are an individual and you should partner with someone that moves at approximately the same pace as you do. Someone a little faster can help to get you going faster, but too fast can hurt you if you are not ready to go faster. You must learn to listen to your body and learn not to overtrain.

Getting with a running club will help you to meet many people and you can have the opportunity to run with the ones that run at your pace and hopefully you can graduate to run with faster runners. Just keep in mind that you want to advance slowly.

HEART RATE

For most beginners, a heart rate monitor is not required. When you become a veteran runner, you can try the heart rate monitor. There are two methods of training: pace based and effort (heart rate) based. The old tried-and-true method is to know your current running or walking pace and slowly increase that pace. For example, if you are a walker, you should try to get to where you are walking at a fifteen-minute pace per mile. That is four miles per hour—the pace you want if you plan on walking a marathon or half marathon. Then you will not get picked up by the bus which gathers slow participants.

Heart rate-based training is more scientific and better for your progress because you train at the intensity that your body allows. Unfortunately, being precise requires costly equipment. You will need a heart rate monitor. You will have to check your resting heart rate and calculate your maximum heart rate. There are many new timepieces available on the market that will tell how far you have run, at what pace, what percentage of your maximum heart rate you are running at, etc. It is a good idea to have a target heart rate calculator. You can download this nomogram at www.coachbenson.com/forms.

You will need to know your resting heart rate. Measure this when you wake naturally (no alarm), do it three (3) days, and then take the average of the three readings. You need to count the number of beats for sixty (60) seconds to get the number of beats per minute. This is required to use the nomogram to know the percentage of maximum that you are running at. It is also required to know during training so that you can check every couple of weeks for any radical change to determine if you are overtraining. You measure by placing your index finger and middle finger on your carotid artery on your neck. You can also use the radial artery on your wrist to measure.

Once you know your resting heart rate, you will want to determine your maximum heart rate. You only need your age for the right side of the nomogram (maximum heart rates are already calculated by age). Draw a straight line from your resting heart rate to your maximum heart rate, and then you can see what heart rate you should be running at for any percentage of your max. Even if you do not have a heart rate monitor, you can stop at any time during exercise and check your heart rate manually to get an idea of where you are on the percentage scale.

In your training program, you will want to start running at a very slow rate (60 percent of your maximum heart rate). For up to 85 percent of your max, you are running aerobically (with oxygen). Once you go over 85 percent you are running anaerobically (without oxygen). Anaerobic exercise burns fat, but don't be tempted to start at that pace. You want to build up your muscles slowly to avoid injury. Do not overtrain. A good way to determine if you are overtraining is to know your resting heart rate and check it at least once every two weeks. If you see a significant change, you should take a few days' rest.

FORM

Proper form is running or walking with the body erect and with a slight (one degree) tilt forward at the ankle. Stand erect and feel your weight in the heel of your foot. Lean forward at the ankle just a bit, and you will feel your weight in the middle of your foot. This is the way you should run. You should come down with your entire weight over your foot. Push off with the forward part of your foot and come down on the other foot in the same manner. You run with your hands, and you run *on* your feet. Your hands should be in a straight line forward and back. Your hands should never pass the center of your body. The shoulders should not move back and forth. The shoulder is merely a fulcrum for your hands to move back and forth. Twisting the upper part of your body is a waste of energy, and you need all of your energy to go faster and further. The faster you go, the more your hands will come up, because you are using more energy and working harder.

Remember to never allow your hands to go past the midsection of your chest. Keep your elbows in close to your body. Remain relaxed. Your shoulders and the upper part of your body do not have to move. The shoulder is merely a fulcrum for moving your arms back and forth. I truly believe that if you run with the correct form and do not overtrain, you should be able to train and be injury free. Physical strengthening of the CORE and FEET will help to guarantee this.

DO YOU NEED A COACH?

Having a coach can most certainly make a big difference in how you train and how well you accomplish your goal, whatever it is. Before signing up with someone, be sure your coach is certified and has done a great deal of reading and studying. I recommend RRCA Certification, which is certification for distance runners. RRCA also has continuing education and requires that certified individuals be current with CPR and first aid. Track and field certification is nice to have, but it covers only track work and field work (throwing and jumping). A 5K is long distance for track and field.

Whether your coach is RRCA or USATF certified, I believe that a track workout (see the next section for more on these kinds of workouts) should also be done with a certified coach. One day a week of speed work is important to getting your body accustomed to running (or walking) fast. You will stress your body more doing speed work than when just going for a run, even if it is a long run. A coach will get you moving at a rate that your body should be able to handle. He or she can watch your form and make suggestions on how you can improve. If there is anything that you do not understand about running, your coach should be able to answer or get an answer to your question.

However, when it comes to coaches, many are great runners, and their technique for coaching is, "This is the way I do it, and this is the way you should do it." What they experience just may not hold true for you. For example, you may have a coach who runs a seven-minute mile and who encourages you to do the same. While the encouragement is important, it does not mean you have to keep up with him or her. You may never be capable of running a seven-minute mile—many people can't. But that does not mean you should give up running. You do not even have to give up your coach. Just find someone else with whom to run or walk. Help coach each other.

Whether you are running and/or walking with a coach, a friend, or by yourself, you should not be embarrassed if you have to walk. Each of us is an individual, and we must do what our body tells us to do. Just don't wimp out. The human body likes to be pushed, so keep trying to push it a little at a time. In time, your body will amaze you as to what it can accomplish.

Track Workouts

The track workout is one of the most important workouts you can do every week. I like to see both runners and walkers on the track every week. The standard outdoor track is 400 meters (440 yards), and the two semicircles and two straight portions are each 100 meters long. Four times around a track is a mile. Workouts can consist of 200s, 400s, 800s, 1600s, etc. The more modern rubberized track is preferred, but the old fashioned gravel track still works. If no rubberized track is available and/or no certified coach is available, then a soft, flat surface (as soft as possible) should be marked out with quarter-mile sections for a total of one mile. This course can be used, but I do not recommend that you practice too often at anything near 100 percent of your maximum heart rate. Stay down under 85 percent.

An example of a workout is a warm-up (generally a walk or jog of half mile or one mile) and then 4X400 with a 200 recovery. Then I like to see fast sprints—2X100—followed by a cool down. (I like to see at least a mile walk or jog for a cool down.) Remember that you will be doing 4X400s, so start slow and increase your pace with each additional 400. This is called negative splits. The 200 recovery can be taken at an easy jog or walk. Take enough time to bring your heart rate down to normal (indicated by normal breathing). The goal of track workouts (over time) is to increase pace and reduce your recovery time.

I sometimes have a group run, and I get out in the middle of the track and blow a whistle every thirty seconds (or twenty-nine, twenty-eight, etc.) so that my trainees can learn how to pace themselves. Thirty seconds per 100 meters is equivalent to an eight (8) minute per mile pace. Each added or subtracted second is equal to 16 seconds per mile. Do the arithmetic. My trainees can be any age, either sex, and of varied athletic ability. I try to get them grouped together by athletic ability to train together when teaching how to pace themselves. The slower individuals have to push a bit harder to be at the right place when the whistle blows, and the faster ones have to slow down. Learning to pace yourself is just as important as running faster. Whether you are alone or with a group, you should be trying to get a little bit faster every week, even if it is by just one second. A monthly mile time trial is also a good idea to let you know if you are improving. The time trial should be done on your first visit to the track and then done each month thereafter. Either you or your coach should keep a record.

I like to see my walkers out there trying to run a little more each week. Even two or three steps more each week is great. Keep a record of what you do, and you will be amazed when you look back after several months. Remember that the human body likes to be pushed, as long as the pushing is done slowly. A hard workout day should be followed by an easy day. Easy days are run or walked about one minute slower per mile than hard days. All workouts should *not* be done at more than 80 to 85 percent (go back to your nomogram and check where you are at) effort unless you are on a rubberized track. I recommend that you only go all out at 100 percent effort on a rubberized track or in a race. **Listen to your body**.

The Long Run

Long, slow runs or walks are essential, whether you are training for a marathon or a 5K. In the beginning your pace will be at 60- to 70-percent effort (check your nomogram), and after a few weeks it can be increased to 70 to 80 percent. Periodically check your pulse during workouts to keep yourself at a slow pace. When you start, a long run can be two, three, or four miles. Eventually you will get to ten, twelve, fourteen miles, and more. These long, slow runs teach your body how to handle the build-up of lactic acid.

The harder you work your body the more lactic acid will build up. The long, slow build-up lets your body absorb this acid; teach your body how to breathe and how to get the maximum amount of oxygen your muscles need. This is running aerobically (with oxygen). Oxygen helps your body dissolve lactic acid, and when your body knows how to handle the acid, you can run anaerobically (over 85-percent effort) without developing the burning sensation.

If you are training for a marathon or a half marathon, you will have to increase your pace a little bit as you get closer to your race day. A long run can be ten miles or much more, depending on where you are in your training schedule. Remember that schedules are made to be changed. As you train, you (and your coach) can evaluate where you are and whether your schedule can be increased or backed off. Corrections should be made as you go along in your training. The schedule should be customized for *you*.

There are many schedules on the Internet, and they may work for you. They are very generalized and separated into novice, intermediate, and advanced levels. If this is your only choice, then start with the novice schedule and try it for a while. If it seems to be too easy, then go to the next step.

The long run should depend upon your ability and target goal (a specific event). The long run should increase by 10 percent to 20 percent each week (total weekly mileage should not increase by more than 10 percent). After increasing for four weeks, go back to the mileage you ran three weeks ago. If the schedule calls for ten, twelve, fourteen, and sixteen mile for a four-week period, then it returns to twelve, fourteen, sixteen, and eighteen mile. The next four weeks would start at fourteen miles and go up to twenty miles. Depending on your running experience and the time available for you to train, there may be the possibility to have a ten-mile run (for the half) or a fourteen-mile run (for a marathon) as a base to stay at for extra rest. If you are a new runner, start your training for large events early. For a half marathon, your longest and fastest run should be done two weeks prior to the race. For a full marathon, your longest and fastest run should be done three weeks before the race. Tapering is done after the final long run. Tapering is a very important part of training, and it helps the body rejuvenate itself after the long hard work you have subjected it to. Your schedule will call for cutting back on your mileage. The week before your race, you should run or walk five, four, three, two, and one-mile. Trying to catch up for missed training can cause you to injure yourself. If you are not trained by the time you do your final long run, back off and do the race at a slower pace than you planned. You cannot complete the race at a pace faster than what you have trained.

Let's stop for a moment and think about the long run. If you are new to running and are planning on completing a marathon, consider doing one or two half marathons before tackling a full marathon. I suggest a full year of training before your first half marathon. This year should be spent learning to run with the correct form, doing strengthening exercises to get your body ready for running or walking for three (3) or more hours. Learn to eat properly before, during and after your long run and finally meeting other runners and walkers and developing the frame of mind that will get you accepting this new way of life. After your first or second half marathon you should be ready and excited to start training for six (6) months to do a full marathon.

Tempo Run

A tempo run is running at your 10K pace for at least twenty minutes. This is not for the beginner. Try to start with running at a fast pace for two minutes, at an 85-percent effort, and then build on that. Even walkers should do a fast walk for two minutes and increase the time and pace a little bit each week. Eventually the goal is to get to walking or running as fast as you can for twenty minutes. Remember to do a warm-up before your workout and a cool down after.

I like to alternate each week from the tempo run to hill running. So one week you do tempo and the next week you do hills. The hills do not have to be mountains. Find a park or a golf course that has some hills on grass. The soft grass surface is easiest on your body. Raise your knees high and run up hard. Walk down and then repeat. One is probably enough the first time. Do a little more each time you do hills. Listen to your body. After several weeks you can run back down. Let the hill take you. Do not lean back and try to apply the brakes. As long as it is not to long or steep a hill You will not roll over. Try it once to get the hang of it. Do not lean back. You can hurt your back by coming down on your heels and trying to slow down.

Easy Run

The easy run is just that. Initially, "running easy" means just running or walking slower than you usually do. When you know what your race pace is, then "easy" means running or walking one to two minutes per mile slower than your race pace. Run easy for a distance that is half of what you are running for your long run that week. If your long run is four miles, then you will run two miles easy. If your long run is twenty miles, then you will run ten miles easy. This run is just to let your body know that you can run easy and to let it know that you are still running or walking every week.

The easy run is a fun run to keep your body moving. Remember that running is fun. You are out there generally working your butt off. One day a week you get to just relax and learn to have a nice easy run that hopefully will make you want to run and/or walk for the rest of your life.

Cross Training

Running uses specific muscles, and to maintain a good overall body, you should work every muscle you have. Cross training is anything that is exercise with *no* impact. Swimming is one of the best things that you can do, because you use every muscle and joint in your body. Not only is it non-impact, but it is floating in water, which supports your entire weight. Water jogging is another useful exercise. Buy a flotation belt, get into the deep end of a pool, and start a jogging motion. This can be tiring and boring, so build up slowly and plan beforehand on what you will be thinking of while you are doing this. You can get all your problems solved while jogging in the water. Water jogging is an excellent way to continue training if you have an injury. Other cross training exercises are cycling (indoor or out), elliptical trainers, stairs, light weights, rollerblading, yoga, and Pilates, among others. Muscle enhancement training can include weight training, but here you want to concentrate on strength. Even sex is a good non-impact, calorie-burning exercise if you can manage to do it for at least an hour.

As part of your cross training, consider exercising your mind as well. Pick up a few books on kinesiology. This is basically the biology or biomechanics of running. This is definitely for the runner who wants to get much better. One great text is *Explosive Running* by Michael Yessis, PhD.

For runners, strengthening the body from the waist to the bottom of the feet, is essential to help ward off injuries. Walking barefoot and slow jogging on a soft surface will help to strengthen the feet and legs. If beach sand or a smooth grass surface is available, be sure to use it as often as possible. At the gym use a BOSU to do a dance (barefoot) and move the feet, ankles, knees and hips. Use the BOSU or a ball behind your lower back to do sit up crunches.

Rest

A rest day is just as important as one of your workout days. Rest days give the body time to heal and recuperate from the beating you have been giving it. This means that you should *not* do anything strenuous like play tennis, mow the lawn, etc. Learn to hear the signs that your body sends you. Listen to your body. Not only should you have one day of rest, but you should plan on getting a good night's sleep every night of the week. After a hard running workout at the track, you should sleep much better. The long run will also tire you out enough to help you sleep.

You'll also want to get good sleep because most races, particularly in warm climates, start at 6 or 7 am, before the sun comes up. If you are not accustomed to rising early, you should start practicing this. Remember the old adage, "early to bed and early to rise makes a man healthy, wealthy, and wise." You are getting into a new way of life, one that is healthy and will make you live longer. Take advantage of the situation and make the most of it. You will be meeting new, healthy, fun-loving people.

To Review

- Decide on using either pace-based or effort-based running.
- Get a runner's watch. Either basic, to know your time, or more expensive, to check your heart rate, distance, pace, etc.

- Determine your resting heart rate range. This can be done without a heart rate monitor.
- Establish the proper running form.
- Consider working with a coach.
- Avoid overtraining. Follow your schedule (run 4 days, cross train 2 days, and rest one day).
- Work on a track when you can. (Rubberized if available.)
- Vary your workouts – If you must vary the days of your schedule remember hard then easy.
- Remember to rest.

Chapter Three
Preparing Mentally

Goals

Whether it is in a race or simply training, have a goal. That goal should keep you going. Many experienced runners have a plan for what they want to accomplish in every run, such as shaving a few seconds off their time or running a little farther. As a beginner, your goal may be to walk a little less and run a little more each time you go out.

By setting a realistic goal, you have the best opportunity to succeed and meet the challenge you set for yourself. Maybe you want to join a running club or organization where you can find friends to run or walk with. Set specific appointments to meet a group or a friend—you will not want to break these appointments, and it will make you want to get up and work out. The more you continue on your schedule, the more you will not want to miss a day. You will probably get to the point where if you miss a day you feel as if you left something out of your life.

The more goals you reach, the more addictive running and walking can become, but it is a great addiction. It is an addiction that makes you feel good and happy with your way of life. Each successive achievement not only makes you feel better about yourself, but it also helps you maintain a positive outlook. For example, a morning run before your normal daily schedule will make you feel as though the day was made just for you. You may initially be more tired, but in a fairly short time you will find that you are invigorated and feeling much healthier.

Maybe better health is your long-term goal. To get there, start by setting a short-term goal or a goal you can easily achieve. This really depends on each individual. Did you run in high school or college? Are you a runner or a walker? How old are you? How healthy are you? These are some of the things that must determine what your goal is. Do not try to set your goal based on some impossible dream. Start off easy and grow into it. You can always change your goal as you continue to train.

Do not try to set your goal based on a friend's goal. This may push you to the point of injury—play it safe rather than sorry. Running and walking is fun, and you are sure to improve with time. You may want to be competitive, but in the beginning, be cool. Your new, healthy body will be the best reward you can give yourself.

One goal is to have a schedule that fits your way of running or walking. The schedule can be changed during your training if you improve enough to make the schedule harder. If you have a coach, do not change your schedule without discussing it with him or her.

Perhaps you are working toward a goal and decide (assuming this decision is from your training rather than fear) that a long run is too long or a track workout is too hard. As long as you have the proper running form down pat, you should probably push yourself harder. Part of positive thinking and part of improving yourself is pushing yourself. That's how you reach your goal.

Unfortunately, there are also those who are not as advanced as they think and should pull back to match their capability. It takes a good coach with experience to tell the difference, but as an individual you should know your body and your capability better than anyone else. Just don't give up on your goals.

Consider setting up a training schedule with specific days set as goal days. There are hundreds of schedules available online. RRCA, *Runner's World*, and most organized marathons offer training schedules on their Web site. An Internet search for any one of these will give you a schedule to train with. Most schedules on the Internet are set up for novice, intermediate, and advanced levels, and these levels can probably cover many runners. Before going off and starting with any schedule, try to find someone who is qualified to check out your running form. Start with the novice or intermediate schedule even if you have been running for some time. After a few weeks of using that schedule, seek advice from a coach, a friend with running experience, a local running store, or a local running club. If you are still in the novice stage, do not continue running without knowing you are running properly. Advancing too fast can lead to injury.

I believe that each runner should have a personalized schedule to fit his or her capabilities. I give each of my trainees a calendar with a schedule made specifically for them. My schedules will have four days of running/walking. The first day of each week is a long run, and I consider what a long run would be for the particular runner's capability. Say a runner has been running for a while and can run eight miles without stopping. Their schedule's long run would start at eight miles, increase to ten the next week, then twelve, and then fourteen. After four weeks the schedule would revert back three weeks and start at ten miles, rising to twelve, fourteen, and then sixteen miles. The amount of time to your chosen event is an important factor in your schedule. I suggest six (6) months of training. For having reached the end of the first four weeks, I suggest a celebration. It's a goal along the way.

Thinking Positive

Most people will never be world-class runners. However, you should not let that prevent you from enjoying the experience of being a good social runner. Eventually you will find that you get the runner's high, and you will also discover that your only real competitor is you.

So get your head on straight. Think positive. A positive frame of mind is very important to how well you run or walk.

Think about it: if you go out there and keep telling yourself how miserable running makes you feel, you are going to have a terrible time. But if you keep telling yourself that every run makes you feel stronger and every day makes you feel healthier, then you are going to enjoy yourself. That is why you should be concentrating on what you are doing when you run.

It also helps to have a mantra. Develop a phrase that you can repeat to yourself to keep you going. During a race you could say, "I have trained hard, and I can do this." During a training run you could say, "I'm going to show my coach that I can kick my own butt" or "I am strong; I am healthy." Make up something that suits your personality and repeat it over and over. Remember to make sure it is something positive. I remember in my training for running hills, I yelled out "charge the hill" over and over again. This helped me get over many hills in a much easier way than just struggling without saying anything.

Perhaps you need a running or walking partner. Not only can you hold each other accountable for getting out there, but you can also remind each other to think positive when any negative thoughts start to creep in. If you don't have someone to run with already, do an Internet search for running clubs in your area. They should be able to help you find other runners at your pace.

Always remember to listen to your body and think positive.

TO REVIEW

- Set short, medium, and long-term goals.
- Make sure your goals are appropriate for you.
- Revise your goals as necessary.
- Create a schedule and stick to it.
- Think positive.
- Develop a mantra.

Part 2

Taking Off

Chapter Four
Training

In my mind, running has always been a very individual sport. The old-fashioned method was to train by yourself and go into a race trying to beat everyone in front of you. Now, with running and walking being a more universal exercise rather than solely a competition among elite runners, there is more friendship and fun involved. But you will still need to train to become a good runner, especially if you decide to participate in a race. A club, a coach, an experienced partner, or pre-designed schedules from the Internet are great training resources. Whatever training plan you use, you must make the commitment and have the determination to stick with it.

Training is not just running. You are an individual and you must learn to know your body. Are there any weak parts of your body? Do you have a queasy stomach? Are you a little over weight? Do you have a tendency to get blisters on your feet? Are you injury prone? There are a million questions that only you know the answer to. As a coach, I can't tell you that you should or should not eat before a race or a long run. I can tell you what foods are good and which are bad, but only you know what will or will not agree with you. I can tell you that if you will be running for more than about two (2) hours you will have to replenish the glycogen in your body. This means that you can run a 5K race with just some water, but you cannot run a marathon without eating along the way. What to eat and how much is what you learn during training. You may have heard the term "hitting the wall". This means that you run out of energy. I can't tell you when this will happen. You should know your energy level at all points during your training. Exactly what kind of sustenance you require (Gu, bars, beans, etc.) and how long they take to kick in, is something that you must learn during training.

We all have a life to live. There are priorities of earning a living, taking care of a family, or many other commitments that only you can answer to. Is a morning run better than the evening? Which days are best? These are things that each of us have to work out on our own. In most cases, changes to our existing schedule must be made.

Don't let this scare you. Training is tough, but it can be the most fun of your new way of life. Even though running is a very individual sport, you want the social aspects that it has to offer. You can meet some very interesting people and make new friends. You can become a member of the running community and always have someone to run with. Running will give you the best return on investment that you can get out of life. Runners live longer.

THE BASIC SCHEDULE

My schedules include four days of running and one day of rest, with every training session preceded by a warm-up and followed by a cool down. I apply this to all runners and walkers. The running days are the long run, the track workout, the easy run, and the tempo run. The long run helps improve your cardiovascular system and teaches your body how to handle lactic acid buildup because you are pushing your body to go farther. Increase the distance of your long run each week for four weeks. In the fifth week, reduce the distance to that which you ran three weeks prior and start the incremental increases again. Repeat this cycle every fifth week. If you have more than six (6) months in your schedule, then you can have a rest period in the schedule where you can do an easier long run. This can help in the overall effect on your body.

If you are training for your first marathon, you'll want to build up your distance to twenty miles, which is run three weeks before the marathon. I do not suggest running more than twenty miles before your first marathon. Coming across the finish line for your first marathon is a very euphoric feeling, and you do not want to spoil that by having run that distance before. This is the goal that you have set for yourself, so why spoil it? If you have trained well and have done twenty miles, you will surely be able to finish the extra six point two miles. There will be enough adrenalin flowing in your body.

The second running day is the track workout. If at all possible, join a group that does a workout on a rubberized track. This surface is very forgiving, and you can practice running as fast as you can. Even if you are a walker, get to a track and try walking faster or even running a little at a time.

The track is 400 meters (440 yards) long and is a good place to try going faster and seeing your improvement as time goes on. You need a warm-up before your workout and a cool down after. The workout could look like 4X400 with a 200 recovery, and 2X800 with a 400 recovery. This means that you do a 400 fast and then a 200 slow, and then repeat until you have done 4. Next, do 2X800 (twice around the track) with a 400 jog or slow walk. I like to see a 100-meter sprint as the final part of a workout. This sprint will train you for a final kick at the end of a race. I also recommend doing negative splits, so look at what your total workout is and plan ahead so that you can complete the whole thing.

As an example, if you are capable of doing a 2-minute 400, try the first at 2:08, the second at 2:06, etc. until you can do the fourth at 2:00. Remember that you still have 2X800 to do in this workout, so plan accordingly. For a 2-minute 400 you should be doing each 100 meters in 30 seconds. You should be checking your watch each 100 meters (while you are running or walking) to know what your 100 meter time is. For a 2:04, you want each 100 meters to be at 31 seconds. Know your plan before you start.

The other two running days are for the slow run, which is half the distance of your long run, and another day to build up slowly for a tempo run (defined as twenty minutes at a 10K pace). With the tempo run, start slowly and build up to the twenty minutes. Split this fourth day with some hill training to build stamina. The hill does not have to be big; just run up, raising your legs as high as you can, and then walk down. Repeat this several times. If you split the fourth day, then two days a month will be tempo runs and two days will be hill runs, which I like to see done on a grass surface when possible because grass and rubberized track surfaces reduce impact on joints.

Do not forget the two (2) days of cross training to exercise the muscles not used in running or walking.

The last day is a rest day. But I recommend doing a 5K race once a month. This not only gives you the experience of doing a race, but it will also keep your fast-twitch muscles awake. However, to avoid injury due to overtraining, avoid running hard days back to back. Maintain a hard-to-easy schedule; the exception is the once-a-month 5K race. Remember the hard/easy concept if you must vary the days of your schedule.

ABILITY

Remember when you were a child, and you just could not grow up fast enough? Now you are in the same position with your running or walking program. If you have already been running, then five or even ten miles may not be too much for you. But if you are a true novice, then one mile may be a long distance. If this is the case, start with a walk around the block. Little by little work up to a half mile, then a mile, and so on. Do not be ashamed to walk. Walking beats being a couch potato.

During your training period you want to find out if you are a walker, a combination walk/runner, or a runner. If you are training for a marathon, you will have to complete at least one twenty-mile walk and/or run, so allow yourself at least six months of training. If you are already capable of running a marathon, then you should be doing two or three twenty-mile runs during your training cycle. I still like to maintain a six (6) month cycle for most new runners and especially for walkers. Training can be reduced to 18 weeks for experienced runners. There are exceptions to every rule, but remember I support injury free running and walking.

Just remember that training schedules will vary depending on your ability. Your age, health, strength, and the amount of time you can spend training all affect your ability. That is why it is important to get clearance from your doctor before beginning any exercise program, especially if you are starting from an inactive lifestyle and you are past the age of forty-five.

Generally you want to get to the point of running and/or walking twenty miles each week, total. Some can begin at this point, and others have to work up to this point. When you get to within three months of your marathon, your schedule should have you running and/or walking twenty to thirty miles per week. More advanced runners will have some weeks where they run as much as forty miles. Think about what this means. If you are running and/or walking thirty miles per week for fifty weeks a year, that is fifteen hundred miles a year. That is a fantastic achievement. Go to the head of the class. You have just become an adult in the running community.

Remember that long distance running is not just putting one foot in front of the other. Start early to know or learn what the correct form is. You run WITH your hands; you run ON your feet. Your hands move forward and back. Do not swing your shoulders. Your shoulders are a fulcrum for your moving arms. Your feet should be supporting the weight of your body. Do not land on your heel or toes. Remember that you are airborne when you run. Each time you land on a foot you should be landing with your body over the entire foot. Practice this in front of a full length mirror, running in place. Do not run on a treadmill (dreadmill). When you come down on a moving surface, unless you are moving at precisely the same pace you will get a slight twist. You may not notice this, but eventually this could cause injury.

Overtraining

Training for running requires the same drive and commitment, and a similar learning curve, as learning any new skill. You must learn to know and listen to your body. You cannot drive across the country on one tank of gas, and you cannot complete a marathon without adding fuel to your body. Your body needs rest, and only you will know how much training is enough.

You don't want to be sidelined with an injury due to overtraining (caused by a killer workout or too much running). Consider finding a partner, preferably one that is just a bit faster than you so that he or she makes you work a little harder. The key word is "little." You don't want to get caught up in overtraining to keep up with a partner. If you can't keep up, either find a new partner or make your partner slow down. As your training improves, you may find that you *can* keep up, and that's good.

However, don't try to do too much too fast. A coach can help you prevent overtraining. Overtraining is the curse of running. So many beginners have the idea that if running five miles is good then ten miles should be twice as good. *Wrong*. You should have a schedule that brings you up very slowly. You should never increase your weekly mileage by more than 10 percent, and every four weeks you should back off to where you were three weeks prior. Your body needs time to build up the ability to run many miles.

There are certainly exceptions to this. If you are young and strong, you may get away with overdoing this rule, but most individuals should build up their body to where they have a few thousand miles on their legs before starting to run any way they want to.

Overtraining is where most injuries occur. Even experienced runners become overconfident and foolishly injure themselves. Stress fractures, knee problems, and lower back problems are some of the most frequent running injuries, and these are all mostly due to overtraining and poor form. Overtraining also applies to racing. Most new runners and even walkers will get into a race, start at the front, and go as fast as they can. They soon find that they peter out and have to start slowing down. You should have a plan for every race and stick to it. Your plan should be based on your training. Many people just refuse to do their homework. They think that they can train at a 10 minute pace and then run a 9 minute pace in the race. This is the dreamer. This just does not happen in practice. Your plan should be based on your training pace not what you would *like* to run.

Listening to Your Body

Your training will tell you how fast you can start a race. You should have a plan for every race you enter, and this plan should be based on what you have been doing in your training. Specificity is how you plan your training, and that is how you train for a specific race. If you are training for a marathon, nothing says you can't do a 5K during your training. In fact, I recommend that you do a 5K once a month during your training. Your time for this shorter race is not important. It is merely something that gives you experience in racing and how to pace yourself. Your plan should be to start slow and pick up the pace as your body tells you to.

All runners should always try to increase their speed, even if it is by one second. One example of picking up the pace is doing negative splits for every run that you do. That is, start slow and get faster as your plan tells you. As an example, if you have been training at around a ten-minute pace and you believe that you can break thirty minutes for a 5K race, then your plan might read that you do the first mile at 10:00. Your second mile might be at 9:55. If you are still feeling strong, you might try a 9:45 for the third mile. This will leave you fifteen seconds for the final tenth of a mile, and if you have been practicing sprints, you should be able to come close to thirty minutes for the race. If at first you don't succeed, keep practicing and try again. You will be successful.

As a beginner, you do not need to run more than twenty to thirty miles per week. As you advance and get more miles on your legs, you can very slowly increase your weekly mileage. Check the section on running form and review what you should be doing. The correct running form will enable you to train to get faster. If I am running near you, I may yell for you to straighten your hands or pull your elbows in closer to your body.

During your training, you must learn what your body requires for the best energy and for the best rest to rebuild your muscles. Everyone requires different amounts and types of food and drink that give them the energy needed to complete a task. You must know what your stomach will and will not accept. Are you allergic to anything you may ingest? What energy fluids, bars, gels, etc. help you and keep you going? Do you need to eat before a long run, or can you get all the energy you need during the run with what you eat along the way? If you are a vegetarian, you will need to check your special needs diet. You need some protein, and you will need some fat.

You learn the answers to these questions during training—you will learn what your body needs to perform well. In this way, running will be a joy rather than a chore, and you can and will continue to be active for the rest of your life.

TO REVIEW

- Training takes time—be patient.
- Create a schedule that reflects your abilities and stick to it.
- Use caution to avoid overtraining.
- Learn to listen to your body.

Chapter Five
Stretching & Muscle Enhancement

Stretching

Stretching is the process of putting different parts of the body into a position that will lengthen certain muscles and their surrounding soft tissue. As part of your exercise program you need as flexible a body as you can get. This will help limit discomfort and reduce the possibility of injury during training. Many of you just getting started will be very inflexible, but just as you increased your distance and speed, you can improve your flexibility.

Start slowly with your stretching program, and to avoid injury, warm up your muscles for a few minutes before you do any stretching. Running in place in front of a full length mirror is a great way to warm up for stretching while also improving your running form.

Yoga and Pilates are two exercises that include stretching, and many of the moves learned during classes for these disciplines can be used to stretch every day. You can go online or look in the yellow pages, but I have found that the best way to find a good gym or place for Pilates is to go to the local running store and ask them for a recommendation. They are in contact with any and all running clubs in the area and can get you into the place that is best suited to your requirements.

For our purposes we will be doing static stretches. Static stretching is performed by placing the body into a position whereby the muscle (or group of muscles) to be stretched is under tension. You should feel a pull but not extreme discomfort. Hold each position for ten to thirty seconds.

There is also dynamic stretching. This refers to stretching exercises that are performed with movement. For example, it used to be common practice to perform the butterfly stretch by resting the soles of the feet against each other and bouncing the knees. Because such action was later discovered to carry a greater risk of injury, static stretching for the butterfly stretch is now recommended and considered more effective. But remember, in running you should never overtrain, and in stretching you should never overstretch. Do every stretch slowly, and increase your range of motion a little bit at a time.

Unfortunately, the research (a group in Australia sent out a survey to thousands of coaches around the world) done to date comes up with about 50 percent in favor of and 50 percent against stretching. Both groups, however, consider strength and stamina, with an emphasis on core strength, to be necessary for good health and good running. Most strength exercises also stretch your body. If you stick with sit-up crunches, back exercises, the Pilates, the plank, etc., you can develop a great body and be very capable of being a good runner.

Muscle Enhancement

There are plenty of ways to spend lots of money to help you develop a good, strong body. I have found that most of the exercises you would learn can be done at home with a few inexpensive items (large ball, rope, mat, etc.). The problem is that most of us do not have the drive to do these things on our own. It is nice to have a private coach, a personal trainer in the gym, or anything else that holds us accountable and makes us come to an appointment. If you can afford it, great. If you can't, just remember that all of this information can be found by checking online or going to the library and reading about stretches, Pilates, Yoga, etc.

Most runners and walkers believe that a running shoe takes care of their feet and do not exercise to strengthen their feet. The feet take the brunt of the force in running and walking. It is essential to strengthen the tendons, ligaments, and muscles of the feet. This can be done by walking BAREFOOT. Just like in running, you should walk on a soft surface: in the house on carpet, on the beach sand, or on groomed grass. Strong feet will help you avoid injuries. After walking for several weeks, you can try jogging slowly. More advanced would be to do strides (run hard for about 100 yards and walk back) BAREFOOT.

Many hospitals now offer classes in stretching, Yoga, Pilates, etc. at a very low cost. Just get your head straight and get the job done.

Massage is a stretching of all muscles and a pressing of many pressure points. Thai or shiatsu massage is a technique you should try if you are looking for something that goes one step beyond a standard massage. They are really not anything like a regular massage. There is no oil and no rubbing. You should be dressed comfortably with nothing in your pockets or on your body. Call around to several massage places and ask if they have someone trained in Thai massage. It can be expensive, but it is worth a try if you have a particular spot that hurts. All massage is a nice thing and can help to make you feel better. Though it is costly, you should try it if you can afford it. It is not something that I consider an absolute necessity.

'Fraid Nots, by Tom Drum, is a book on rope-assisted stretching that comes with a rope. The rope makes a small package and can be carried with you in your workout bag. It is a very convenient item to carry when you travel as well. It is an excellent device you can always have with you to stretch after your run. This item is fairly inexpensive and is available in many running stores.

The ball, like the rope, is a useful stretching and workout assistant. Every gym has several of these. The ball is generally about twenty-four inches in diameter and can be blown up very easily. They are not too expensive an item if you want one to use at home, and they can be easily purchased from most stores carrying workout equipment. When purchasing a ball, be sure that a booklet showing how to use it is included. When working with the ball, remember to maintain a neutral spine, and engage your core by using your transverse abdominals to pull your navel in toward your spine. Some example uses are:

- Squats—place the ball between your back and a wall. Lower yourself to a sitting position and then reverse the procedure.
- On your back—lying on your back, hold the ball between your feet. Raise your legs and arms and transfer the ball to your hands. Lay flat, lowering your arms over your head, and then raise up your arms and reverse the procedure.
- Side lifts—Lie on your side with your head resting on your arm. Hold the ball between your ankles. Lift your feet off the floor on exhale, and inhale as you to lower your feet. Do not let your feet touch the floor.
- Rolling with the ball—Lie face up on the ball. Holding your abdominals tight, walk forward, allowing the ball to roll along your spine until it is resting under your shoulder blades. Walk back up. Let the ball roll up your spine by itself. Do not crunch up.
- BOSU—an hemisphere with a blue plastic dome. About two feet in diameter with the top of the dome, when inflated, about 10 inches above the surface. Most gyms have several. A great device to stand on (barefoot) and do a dance. Move your feet, ankles,

knees and hips. In time this will strengthen your body from the waist to the bottom of your feet.

Stay on for at least 10 minutes each time you use this piece of equipment. It is designed as a balance device, but it is not absolutely necessary to use it without holding on to the wall or something. In time you will develop the balance and by then your legs will be stronger. It also can be used for sit up crunches with the dome under the small of your back. This elevates your back above the floor and in this position you are strengthening the upper and lower Abs.

STRETCHING EXAMPLES:

Artwork by Abigail Elakman (my fourteen-year-old granddaughter).

All stretches should be held for ten to thirty seconds. All stretching should be done with a warm body. After your workout you should stretch for twenty to thirty minutes because your body is warm. By doing easy stretches after working out, you cool down and help to bring your heart rate down to normal.

A basic stretch against a wall or column. Place your hands on the wall and bring your feet about 18 to 24 inches back away from the wall. Stretch this way, and then bring one foot in halfway and stretch the rear leg to feel the pull in the hamstring. Then reverse the feet and do the other leg. This can be done after a warm-up to stretch the hamstrings.

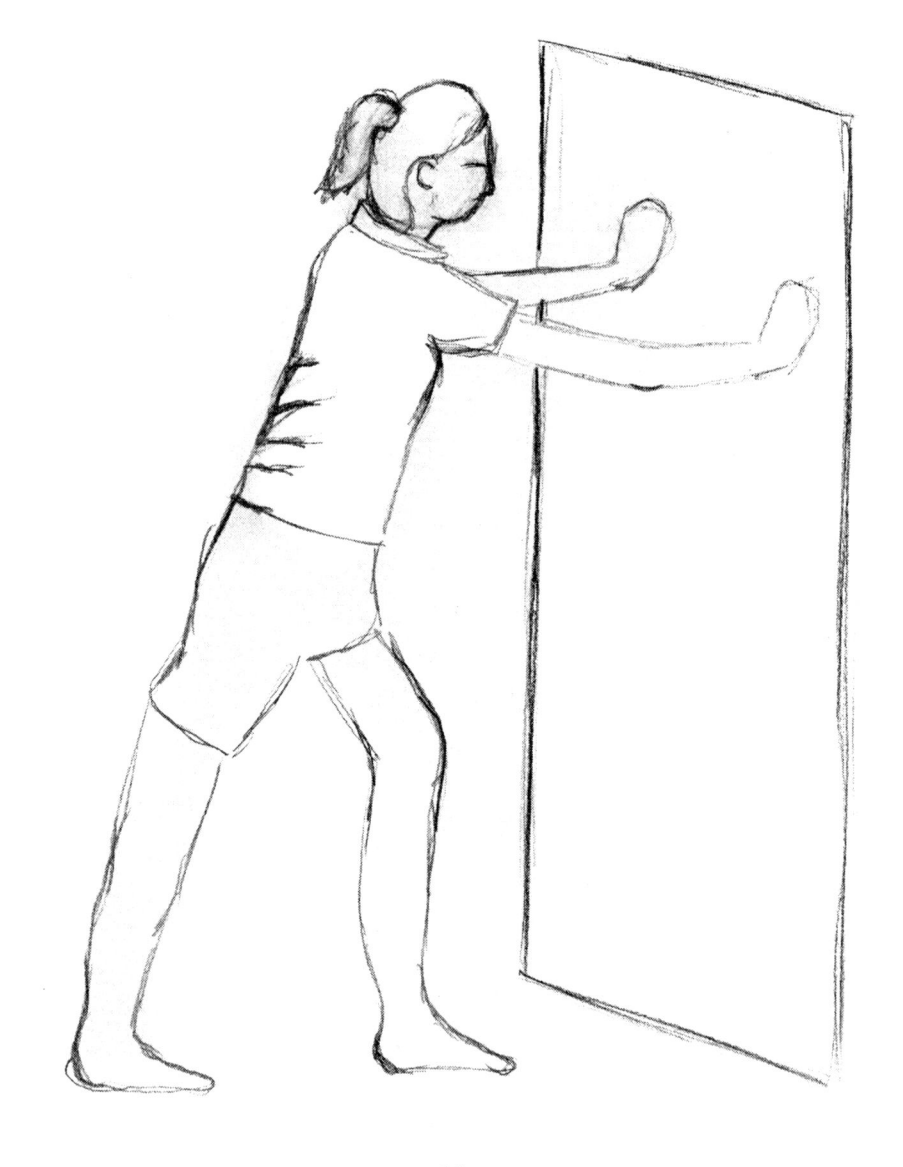

Whole body stretch lying on your back. This is a nice, restful stretch to relax and stretch the back. Resting and stretching on your back can be done at any time. Lie on your back and extend your arms over your head. Keep your toes pointed upward and lengthen your body as much as you can. Pull your gut in and hold for 10 to 20 seconds.

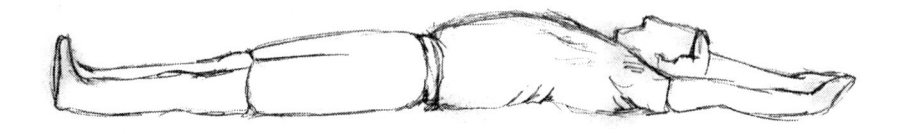

Sitting side-reach stretch. Sit with one leg straight and toes pointing upward. Then bring your other foot onto your knee and let your head fall toward the straight leg. Reach toward the outside of your toes with both hands. Hold for ten seconds. Repeat with the other leg.

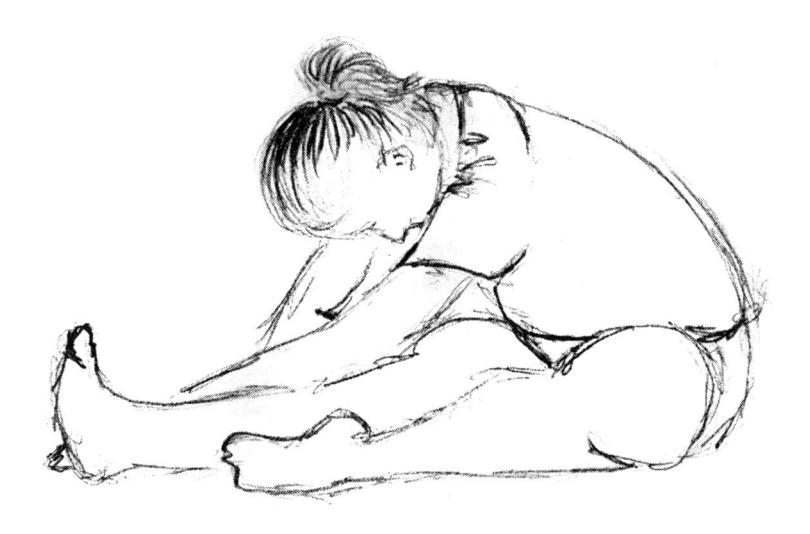

On-elbows stomach stretch. Engage your abdominals when doing this. This position is similar to the one used for strengthening your abdominals where you raise the body and support yourself on your toes and your forearms. That would be called "the plank" in Yoga.

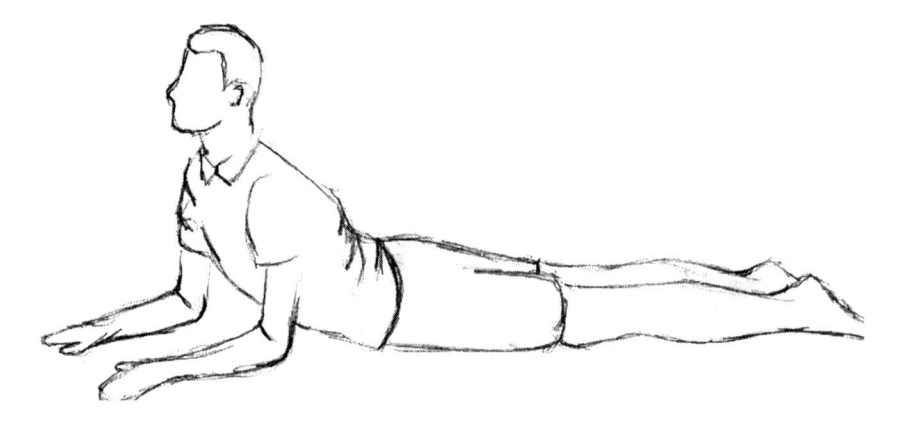

Lying leg-resting buttocks stretch. Lie on your back and slightly bend one leg. Raise your other foot up onto your bent leg and rest it on your thigh. Then reach forward, hold below your knee, and pull towards you. Repeat with the other leg.

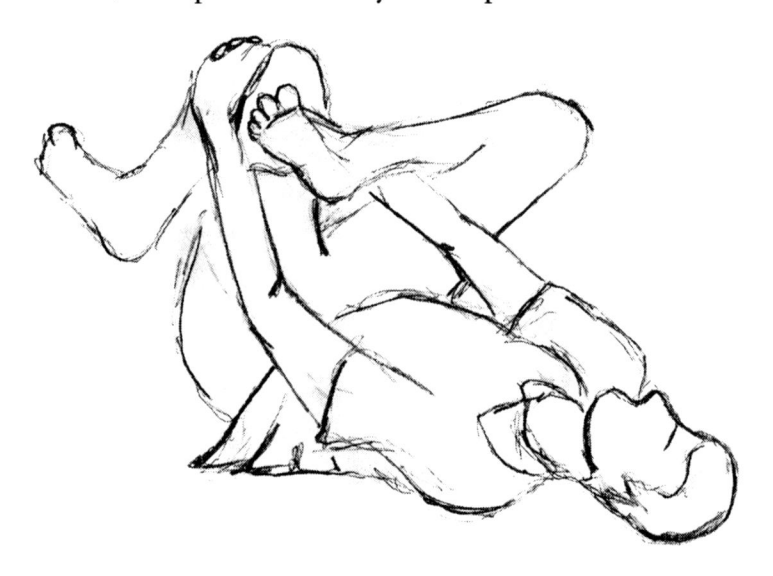

Standing toe-down hamstring stretch. Stand with one knee bent and the other leg straight out in front. Point your toes towards the ground and lean forward. Keep your back straight and rest your hands on your bent knee. Repeat with the other leg.

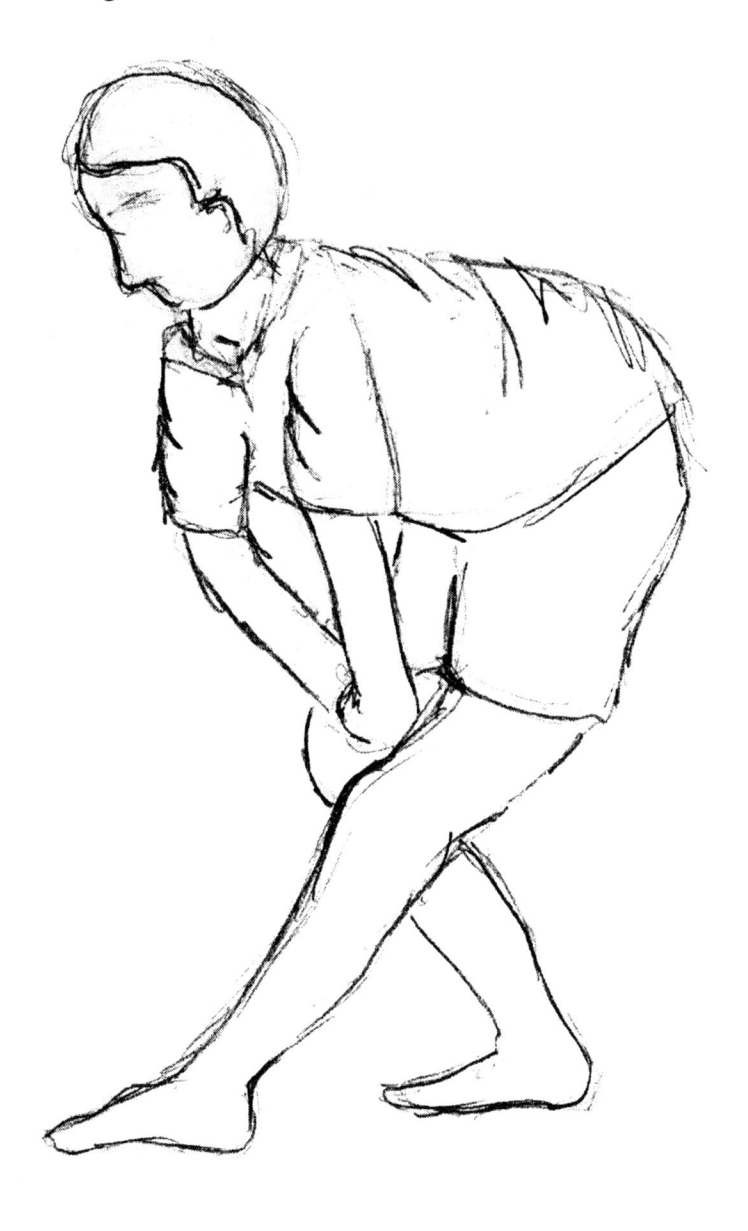

Kneeling face-down adductor stretch. Kneel face down with your knees and toes facing out. Lean forward and let your knees move outwards.

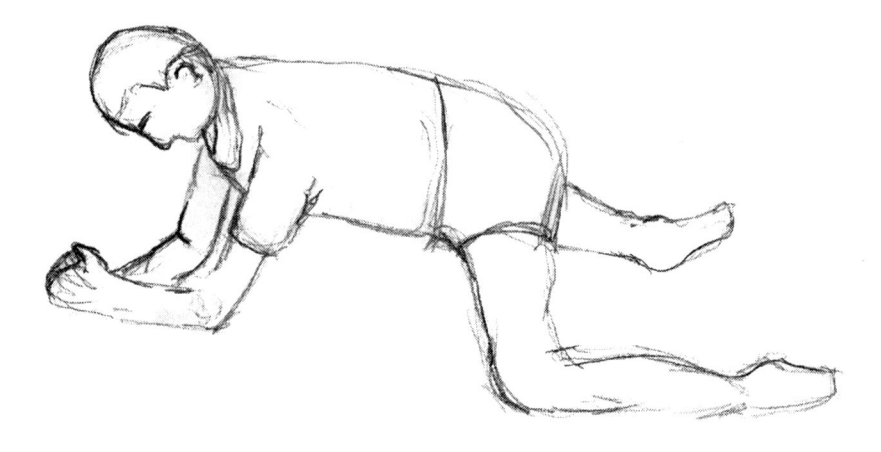

Standing leg-cross abductor stretch. Stand upright and cross one foot behind the other. Lean towards the foot that is behind the other. Repeat with the other leg.

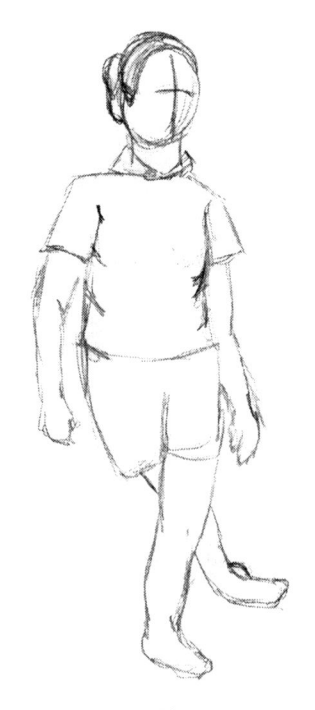

Standing toe-up calf stretch. Stand with one knee bent and the other straight out in front. Point your toes up and lean forward. Keep your back straight and rest your hands on your bent knee. Repeat with the other leg.

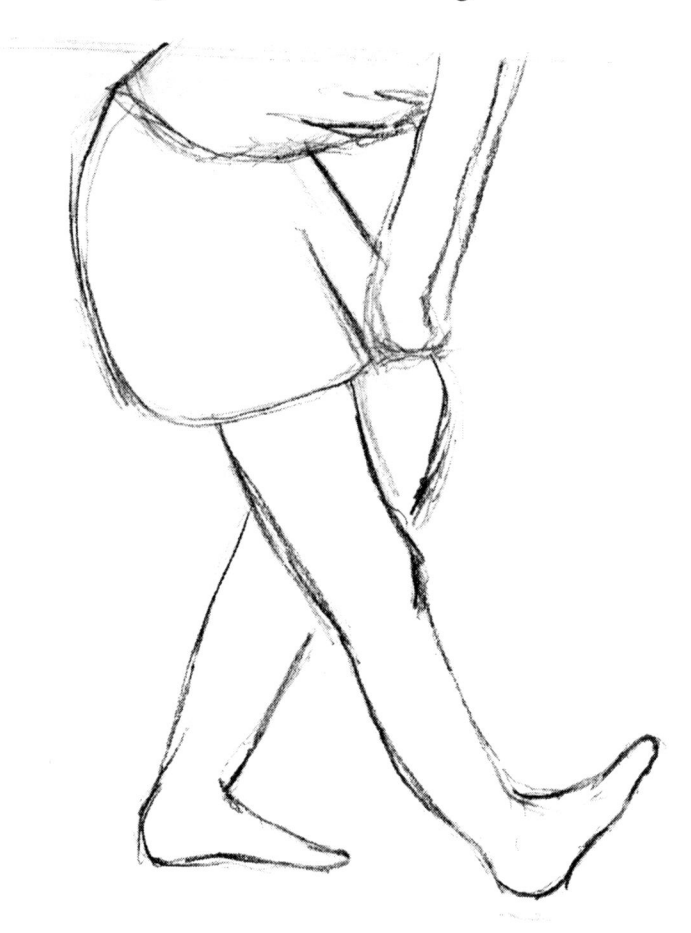

Standing heel-back calf stretch. Stand upright and take a big step backwards with one foot. Keep your back leg straight and your toes pointed forward, and push your heel to the ground. Repeat with the other leg.

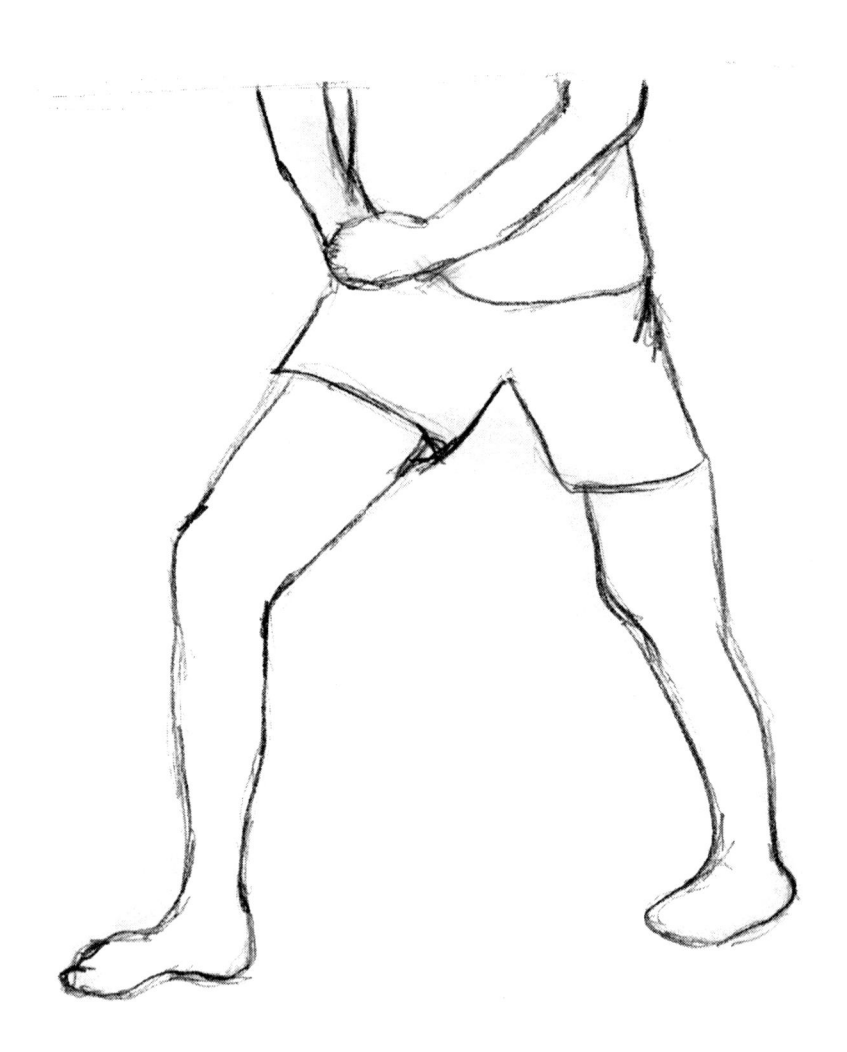

Stepping Forward

Double kneeling shin stretch. Sit with your knees and feet flat on the ground. Sit back on your ankles and keep your knees together. Place your hands next to your knees and slowly lean back while raising your knees off the ground.

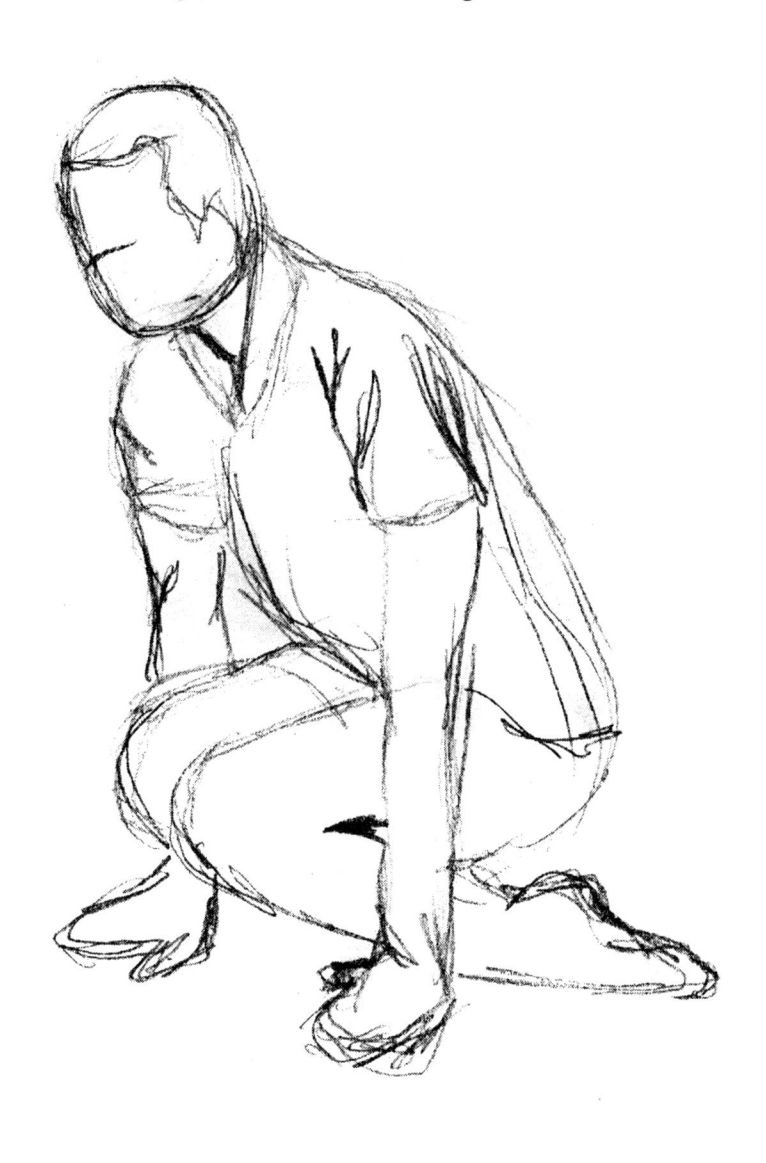

Muscle Enhancement Examples

While you are doing muscle strengthening, you are also stretching your body. Muscle enhancement exercises will condition and improve muscles. They should not be performed on your cross training day. Also, if you choose to use weights you should use them on alternate days, not consecutively. Muscles need time to rest and rebuild.

Cat-cow stretch. Start from your hands and knees. First, round your back up to the sky. Hold, and then arch your back with your head up.
    Stretches—abdominals and torso
    Strengthens—abdominals, neck, front and back of torso

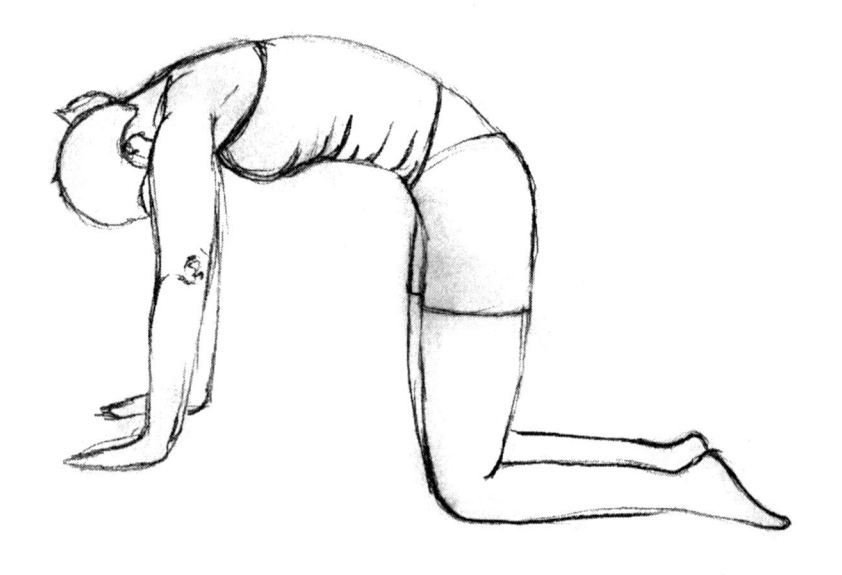

Balancing half moon. From a wide stance, raise your back leg to the height of your hip. Bring your back hand to your hip, with the fingertips of your front hand on the floor, directly under the front shoulder. If comfortable, reach your back (top) arm to the sky. Stay focused. If balanced, look up to the top hand. Switch sides.

Stretches—hamstrings

Strengthens—obliques and adductors

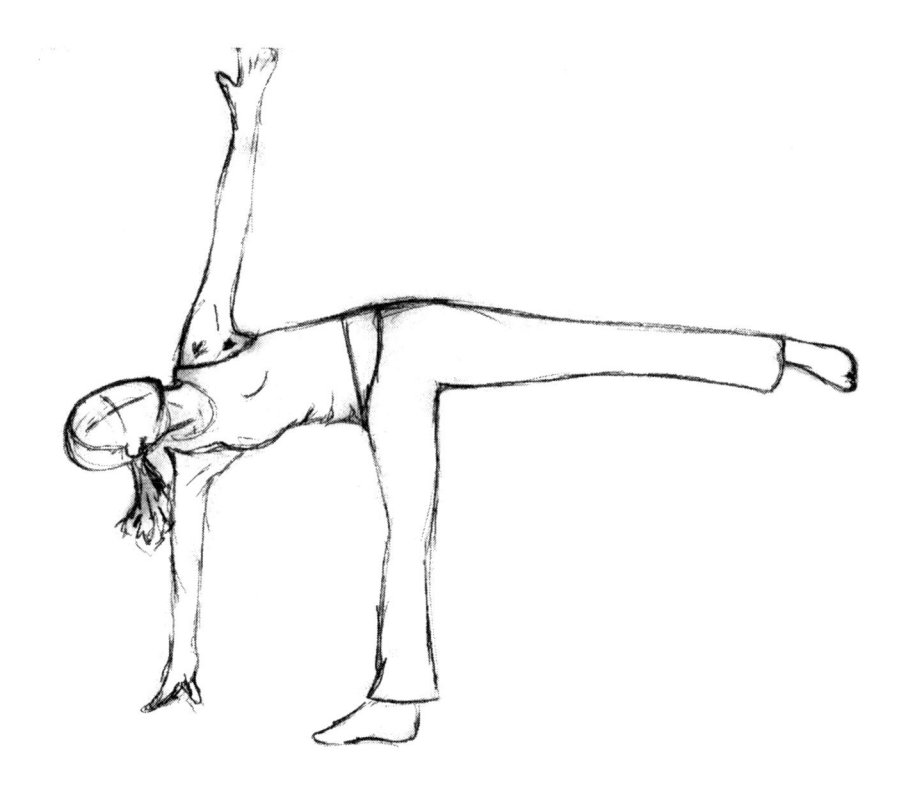

Superman. Lie down on your stomach. Extend your arms forward with your legs straight back. Lift your arms and legs. Lift and stretch your limbs away from your torso. Modify by bringing your arms down to your sides.

    Stretches—front of the body

    Strengthens—back of the body

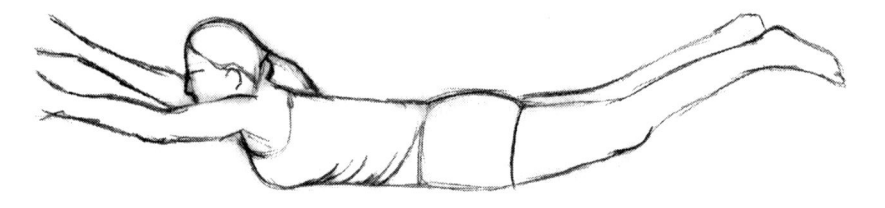

Spinal balance. From the hands and knees, extend one arm and the opposite leg parallel to the floor. Engage your abdominal muscles, keeping a straight spine. Lengthen the extended arm and leg on each exhalation. Hold and then switch sides.

    Stretches—back muscles

    Strengthens—back muscles

    Advanced—Raise foot and balance on knee. Form one straight line from fingertip to toe

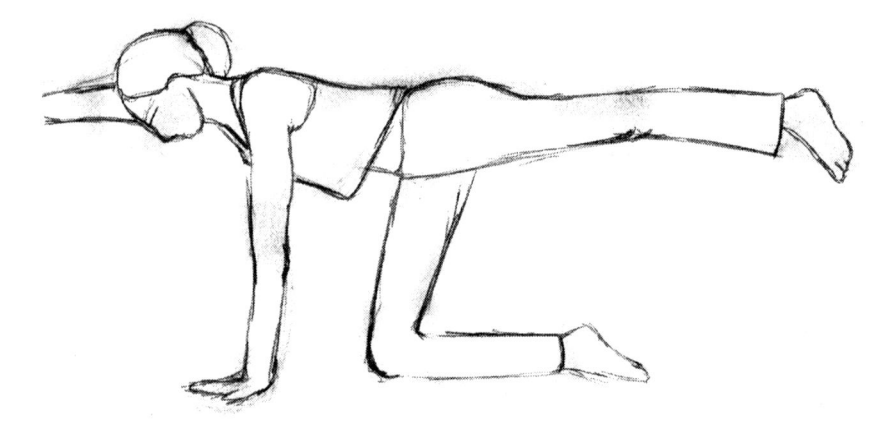

Yoga stretch. Stand with your feet wide apart, one in front of the other. Point your front toes straight ahead, turn in your back toes slightly. Extend your arms out at shoulder height. Bend your front knee and keep your hips level.

Look forward at your hand in front of you. Keep the fingers relaxed. Keep your upper body lifted as you descend into the stretch. Do not let your bent knee fall inward or outward. Keep it bent at a ninety-degree angle, or as close as possible. Tuck your tail bone. Tighten your abs. Watch your knee-to-ankle alignment so that your knee never goes past your toes. Hold and then switch sides.

Stretches—chest to adductors

Strengthens—quads to glutes

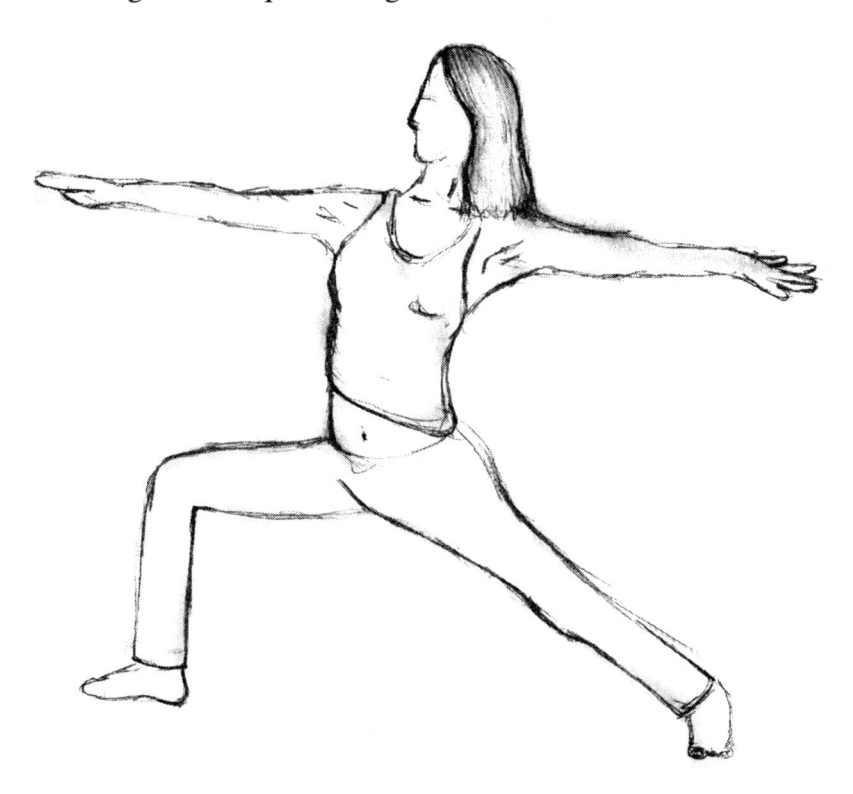

The chair. As if you are sitting in a chair, bend your knees and drop your buttocks. Push your tailbone back. Lift your chest to the sky. Lift your arms parallel to the floor, elbows slightly bent. Keep your knees behind your toes.

Stretches—arms, legs, and back
Strengthens—quads and glutes

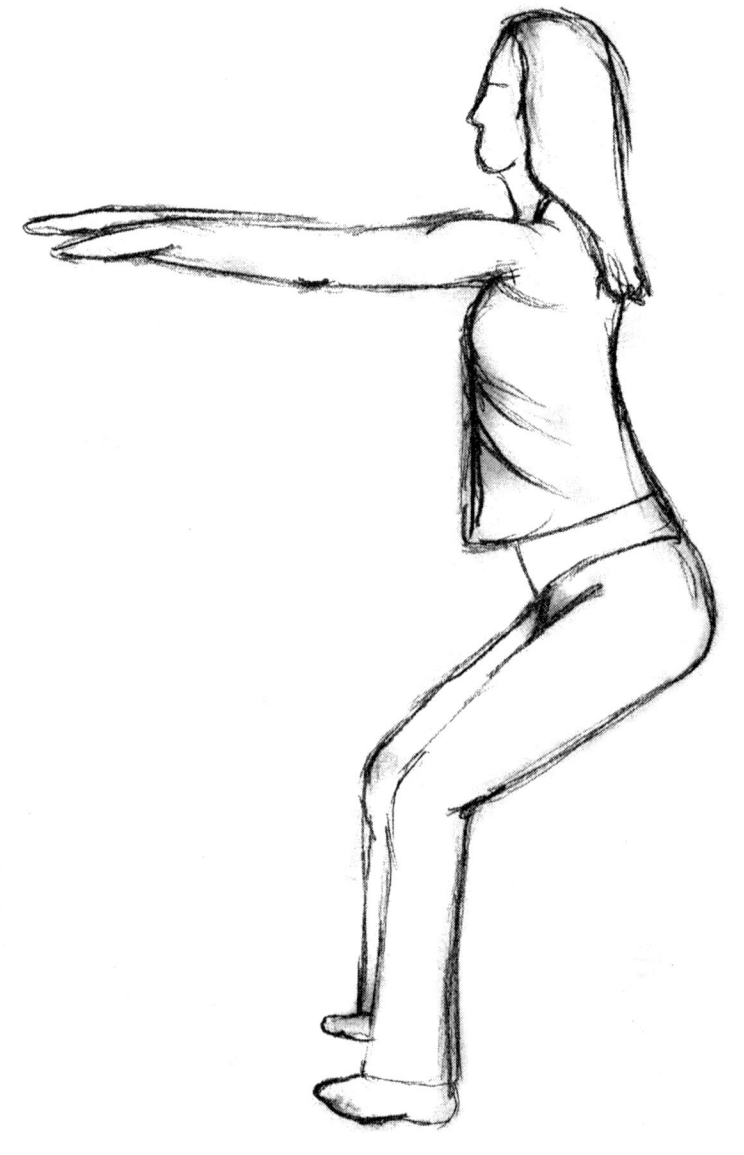

Leg raise. Lie back and support yourself on your elbows. Raise your left leg up about one or two feet with your toes pointed out. Hold for a count of twenty. Repeat with the same leg with toes pointed back toward your head. Repeat with right leg.

   Stretches—calves
   Strengthens—legs and core

   Advanced—Add leg weights.

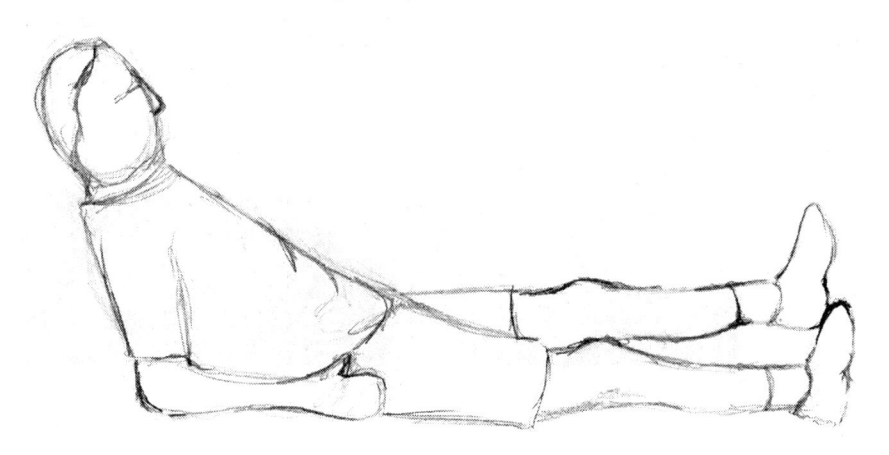

Sit-up crunches. Lie on your back with your feet pulled in close to your butt. Place your hands on the side of your head. Look straight up and do not bend your neck. Tighten your stomach and hold for a count of ten. Work up to repeating one hundred times.

Stretches—abs

Strengthens—abs (this strengthens upper abs only)

Look straight up

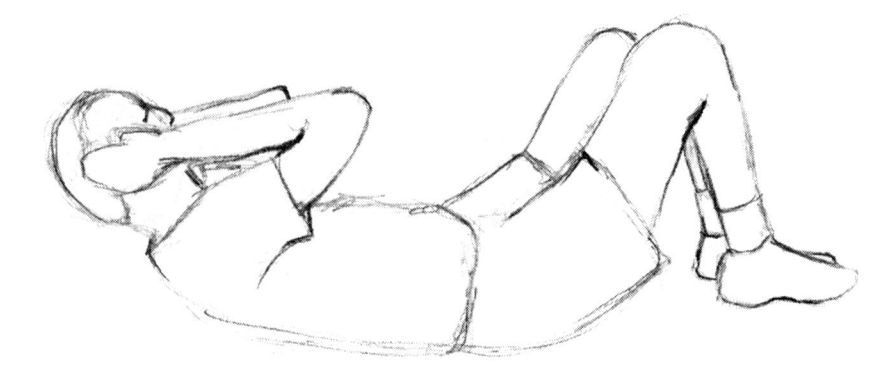

Pilates hundred. Lie on your back. Raise your legs (as high as possible, you'll go higher in time). Raise your head, chin to chest, and stretch your arms out in front of you. Pump your arms up and down five times while breathing in and five times while breathing out. That's one! Repeat ten times (Pilates hundred). Place your hands under your knees and raise elbows. Keep your head forward and push your feet out to a sitting position. Repeat three times.

Stretches—abs

Strengthens—upper and lower abs

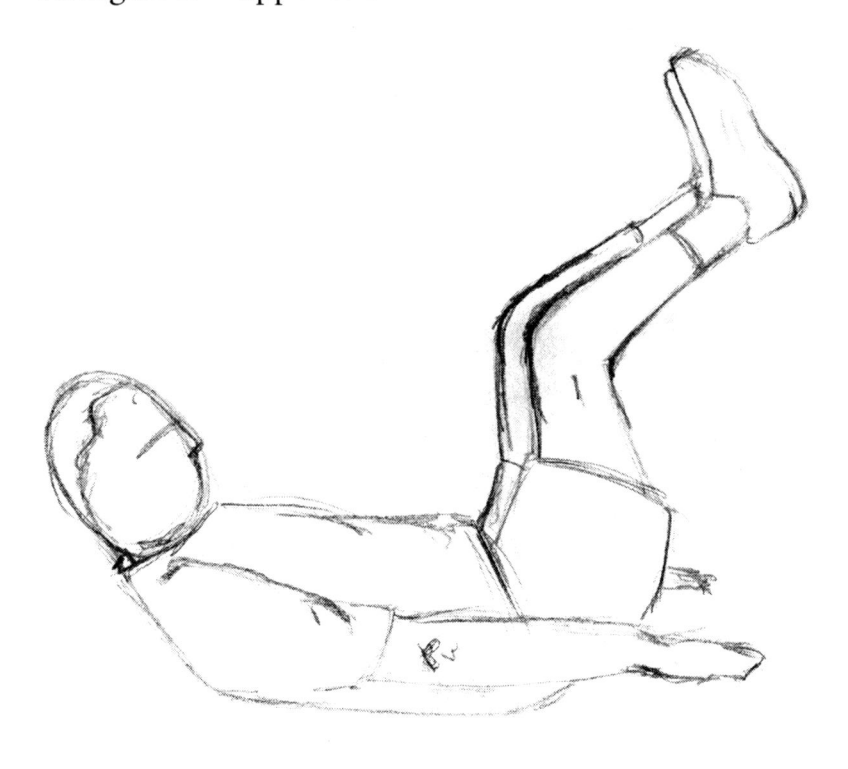

Plank. Get on your elbows and toes. Engage your abdominals and squeeze your butt. Hold this position for as long as you can without overstraining. Slowly, over time, build up to two to three minutes.

Advanced—Raise one leg off the floor and hold the position. Alternate to the other leg.

Side plank. Left side, then right side.

Strengthens—hamstrings, quads, glutes, abs, and back

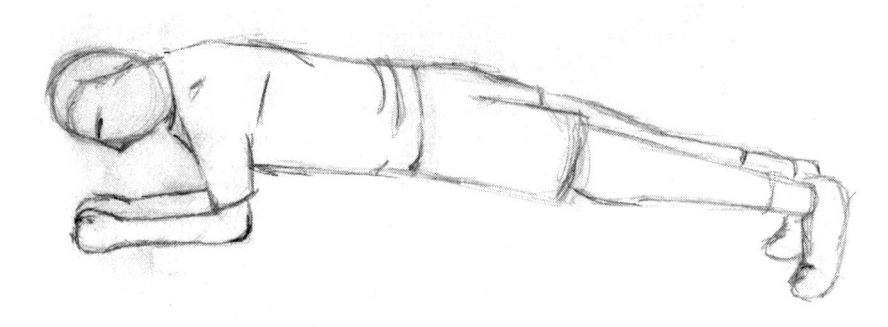

To Review

- Warm up before stretching.
- Perform static stretches and hold them for ten to thirty seconds.
- Develop and maintain flexibility and core strength.
- Find a friend to work out with.
- Training doesn't have to be expensive.
- Core strengthening is just as important as running.
- Strengthen feet by walking and jogging barefoot.

Chapter Six
Nutrition

Eating! One of my favorite subjects. I hate the word *diet*—it should be removed from the English language, along with diet foods and diet drinks. Eating properly should become a way of life. Reduce your fat (especially saturated fats) and sugar intake; learn to live on fruits, vegetables, grains (and other complex carbohydrates), and some protein. Learn to read the labels on all food that you eat and then come up with a method of eating that best fits your way of life.

One technique is grazing, which means eating six to eight small meals a day. This sometimes interferes with the American way of life where people sit down to meals as a family, but it is very important to learn not to stuff yourself. If you are going to eat as a family or eat out, then realize that even though there are children starving elsewhere in the world, you do not have to eat everything on your plate.

CALORIES

Excess calories can add weight. Think in terms of the basic formula: calories taken in must equal the calories burned up in order to maintain your weight. If you want to lose weight, you must burn more calories than you take in. Remember that 3500 calories equals one pound of fat.

Now, I understand that nobody's perfect. Don't feel guilty when you cheat (dessert or sweets, etc.). Just try hard to do it less frequently. Some people cheat only on Sunday. Other people use Monday as a fast day and consume only fresh fruit, fruit juice, and water. Try to come up with a healthy method that fits your way of life. No matter what, it is important that you read the labels on any foods you eat, checking for the ingredients and amounts of fat, protein, sugar, etc.

Fat and sugar make most foods taste good. Sneaky manufacturers remove one of these and double the amount of the other to make sure it still tastes good. Be careful of fat-free or sugar-free labels on packages.

CARBOHYDRATES

As a runner or walker, you need to eat complex carbohydrates to supply the glycogen that you need for fuel. Complex carbohydrates are grains, fruits, and vegetables. Try to stick with whole wheat grains, green and orange vegetables, and fruits of all types. If you have a weight problem, eat your grains in the daytime (so that you can work them off as you do work or exert energy). Eating too much pasta, breads, etc. at night will turn to fat as you sleep and add weight. The body converts carbohydrates into glycogen, which is a sugar and gives you the energy required to run. The night before a hard workout or long race, you should load up on high-fiber carbohydrates. Broccoli is one of the best meals the night before a marathon or a hard workout. High fiber foods are good for you, but if you have not eaten much fiber in the past they can cause constipation. Try adding high fiber foods (green and yellow vegetables and whole grains) to your diet little by little.

Carbohydrates must be broken down into simple sugars and then enter the bloodstream as glucose. The glucose then stimulates insulin, which the body produces to make sure that you do not get too much sugar in your system. Fiber cannot be broken down into simple sugars and has no effect on insulin. Vegetables (such as broccoli) are high in fiber, and the insulin production due to their intake is minimal. Carbohydrates with no or little fiber (such as standard pasta) will stimulate the production of insulin. As a healthy runner and/or walker, you should not have to worry about diabetes; you do not need the insulin.

The glycemic index measures the entry rates of various carbohydrate sources into the bloodstream. The glycemic load, which is a reflection of carbohydrate content, is even more important in determining the insulin output of a meal. One cup of regular pasta and one cup of broccoli have approximately the same glycemic index, but the glycemic load for white pasta is more than twenty times as great as that of broccoli.

VITAMINS, MINERALS, AND PROTEIN

In addition to carbohydrates, it's also important to consume an appropriate amount of vitamins and minerals. For example, runners generally have to avoid muscle cramps, and the mineral potassium helps avoid getting these cramps. Bananas are rich in potassium and, thus, very important to runners. In general, bananas are one of the best foods you can eat. They are almost always served at the end of a race. Make sure you eat several bananas every week. Bananas have 450 milligrams of potassium and about 109 calories. An eight-ounce glass of low-sodium V8 juice has about 900 milligrams of potassium and only 50 calories. A baked potato with the skin has 844 milligrams of potassium and 173 calories. If you are trying to lose weight, calories count, but potassium is required for your body. Calcium is another element required for strong bones. No- or low-fat dairy can supply the calcium that you need. No-fat, plain yogurt with some fresh berries or other fruit makes a healthy meal.

In addition, remember that you also need some protein (chicken, fish, and low-fat meat) for muscle regeneration. Fruits and vegetables (raw or lightly steamed), however, should be the mainstay of your daily food intake. If you are a vegan or vegetarian, legumes and soy products are good sources of protein. You also need some fat in your diet (not saturated or trans fat). As a vegetarian you might consider taking fish oil supplement.

Hydration

In real estate they talk about location, location, location. In running and walking we talk about hydration, hydration, hydration. This means that you must drink fluids. In general, plain water is best. Generally about eight glasses of water per day is required, but it really depends upon the temperature, your metabolism, how much you sweat, your size, and several other factors. You are an individual and must determine how much water you need. Just be sure that you get at least something close to eight glasses (about sixty-four ounces) every day. A better gauge of how much to drink is to drink half your weight in ounces. A 100-pound person will need 50 ounces of water a day, and a 200-pound person will need 100 ounces.

Also, having your stomach filled with water will keep you from getting hungry, so it can be a way to control weight. Alcohol and caffeine are diuretics, which remove water from your body, so if you consume either of these you must then drink an equal amount of water to make up for the loss.

Eat well, run hard, and be healthy. That's a great motto to live by.

To Review

- Eat six to eight small meals a day.
- Equal calories consumed and burned maintains weight.
- More calories burned than consumed leads to weight loss.

- Watch for hidden fats and sugars.
- Consume complex carbohydrates that are high in fiber.
- Consume healthy amounts of vitamins and minerals, especially potassium and calcium.
- Remember to eat some protein to rebuild muscles.
- Stay hydrated.

Chapter Seven
Safety Precautions

In almost every race there will be medical people available to take care of you if you need help. On your long training runs, however, you should always try to run with a companion in case either of you needs medical attention, and if possible carry a cell phone. Your cell phone should have an ICE (in case of emergency) contact number or numbers programmed into it.

Heat Illnesses

Caution should be used when temperatures exceed 82.4 degrees Fahrenheit and humidity rises above 60 percent. Running in such conditions can put you at risk for heat illnesses such as dehydration and heatstroke. Avoid dehydration by replacing fluids with six to eight ounces of cool water every fifteen to twenty minutes. The body absorbs cool water faster. Some of the first symptoms of dehydration are thirst, fatigue, and headaches. If you think you are suffering from dehydration, take a break from your training and slowly drink more cool water.

If dehydration is left untreated, it can lead to a far more serious illness: heatstroke. Heatstroke occurs when the body can no longer cool itself. The symptoms of heatstroke include a temperature greater than 104 degrees Fahrenheit; hot, red, and/or dry skin; disorientation; diarrhea; very small pupils; rapid pulse; and unconsciousness. Someone suffering from heatstroke requires immediate medical attention, as untreated heatstroke can be fatal. The body must be cooled down as quickly as possible. Clothing should be removed, damp cloths can be applied, if there is a fan available to create an evaporation effect it should be used, and water should be consumed if possible. If you have been hydrating and feel sluggish or not up to par, get to a cool place as soon as possible. If you really feel bad, get to an emergency room immediately. Whether you are training or in a race, don't try to gut it out. There are other marathons, and it is better to stay alive and have the opportunity to enter another race.

A word about warm, rainy races—you still need to hydrate even though the rain makes it feel cool and you want to finish as soon as possible. More people finish dehydrated in the rain than in any other weather condition. Water on the outside is not the same as water on the inside. I have worked the finish line of many marathons and have seen this first hand.

COLD ILLNESSES

Just as hot weather can cause health issues, so can cold weather. Wear several layers of clothing when you exercise, and have gloves and a hat that can be pulled down over your ears. Be prepared to remove one layer at a time as you warm up. In a race, throw the garment on the side of the road rather than trying to carry it with you. Do not wear beautiful clothes that you will not want to throw away.

Being exposed to severe cold can lead to frostbite, hypothermia (abnormally low body temperature), and heatstroke (abnormally high body temperature). Frostbite is when the skin and underlying tissues freeze. Normally, getting out of the cold and warming the affected area(s) will remedy the situation. However, if numbness persists after warming, medical attention should be sought.

Hypothermia is when more heat escapes the body than can be produced. Symptoms include a temperature less than 95 degrees Fahrenheit, confusion, and fatigue. If someone is suffering from hypothermia, immediate medical attention is needed. While waiting, get the person out of the cold and replace cold, wet clothing with warm, dry clothing. Do not apply direct heat. In serious cases, death can occur.

Although it may sound odd, heatstroke can occur in cold weather. It is important to wear layers, but it is also important that the clothing allow moisture to be removed from the body so that cooling can continue. Being aware of the above issues and other basic first aid can come in handy.

General Safety Tips

During a race or when you are on a training run, you should always be aware that accidents can happen. You could eat something that does not agree with you, you could fall and break something, or you could suddenly get sick. Anything is possible. Always have your cell phone with you, and always be sure that someone knows where you are running, how far you plan to run, and how long you plan to be out running. Your cell phone is much more important than your headset and music.

Running and/or walking is a great deal of fun and can become a source of meeting new friends, maintaining good health practices, maintaining a body that you are happy with that is both flexible and strong, and most important, maintaining a mind that is happy with life. Research has shown that runners live longer. Remember that the best gift you have ever received is the *gift of life* that your parents gave you. You should thank them forever.

To Review

- Stay hydrated and use precautions to avoid dehydration, heatstroke, and other heat and cold illnesses.
- Carry a cell phone with you.
- Let people know your training schedule.
- Run smart; run healthy.
- If possible, run with a friend.

Appendix A

Look into yourself and know why you are doing this.

1. Know yourself and your limitations.
2. Priority time is required. Are you ready to start getting up early? Will you stay with it?
3. Do you have twenty or more hours a week to commit to training?
4. Join a running club and try it out before you commit.
5. Once you commit, you will be doing this for the rest of your life.
6. Some people commit immediately; others take longer.
7. There is a new world out there full of healthy, fun-loving people.

Appendix B
Marathons: What to Expect

Getting competitive can be fun, depending on who you are. My suggestion is that you talk to a certified coach and get some guidance rather than just going off and starting to run faster and longer on your own. Start slow and build up. Do not overtrain. Be sure to stay hydrated. Maintain good, healthy eating habits. Stretch, do core strengthening, strengthen the feet, and keep a good frame of mind—do not get too upset if someone beats you.

Every community has races almost every weekend and sometimes during the week. If you favor half and full marathons, they can be found every weekend somewhere in the world and possibly even close to your location. Visit the local running store—they will have applications and information about races everywhere. They can usually even help you find someone who is doing a race and looking for a person with whom to share a hotel room. The Internet is a good place to find complete listings of races of every type.

Google *Runner's World* and look at the great information that publication has available.

I've done a New Year's Eve run that started at night and a fifty-mile race and relay in Miami that started on Saturday evening and lasted until about 2 AM. Nowadays I think you would be hard pressed to find a race that started later than 10 AM. In South Florida, races usually start at 6 or 7 AM. Races start later in the north, but not at night. It really depends on your lifestyle and what fits best with your schedule. The old adage of "early to bed and early to rise" seems to fit in best with the runner's lifestyle. If you plan on doing a marathon that starts at 6 AM you had better take that into consideration during your training and reset your biological clock. You have to set your own priorities. What's most important to you? Don't just take the attitude that you can't get up early. Try it for a while and see if you can adapt and maybe even enjoy it. When you make new friends and run or walk in the morning, it can open up a whole new world. See what you miss when you don't see the sun rise. Try everything rather than just saying no.

After you do a good number of marathons and have at least two or three thousand miles on your legs, I recommend that you slowly work up to a thirty-mile run prior to your race day. This long run should be at least three weeks before your marathon. Start your taper after your long run. Tapering should be done prior to any marathon or half marathon. For a full marathon you should taper for three weeks, and for a half you should take two weeks. If you are not ready for your race two or three weeks beforehand, then you have not trained properly. Heavy training two or three weeks before your race is not productive. If you are not fully trained by that time, you risk injury by trying to make up time. You would be smart to cancel and schedule another race in the future.

It used to be that you could wait until just before a marathon to register. These days the more popular marathons fill up almost as soon as they open for registration, which means you have to register almost a year in advance to be sure that you can have a number for the race. This is a good thing because then you'll have the time and the motivation required to train for your marathon.

During training, many people like to stick earbuds in their ears and listen to music. This is fine if you are running in a park or somewhere that has no automobile traffic, but if you are running on the road, please play it safe rather than sorry. In road races, iPods and other such items are not permitted. Unfortunately, it is difficult to enforce this rule, but for safety's sake you should not wear earbuds in road races.

Also, know what the race organizers will offer along the course to drink and eat. In a marathon you must replace some of your electrolytes and protein. Sports drinks do this for you, so try several during training and make sure that your stomach likes what you choose. Do not try anything new during a race. If what they offer is not what your stomach will accept, you will have to carry your own supplies with you.

The night before the race, make sure you eat properly. The old method of carbo loading before a marathon with a pasta dinner should be changed to loading up with vegetables (carbohydrates) that are rich in fiber. A dinner of broccoli, sweet potatoes, and cabbage will do more for you during the race (of course this is the way you should have trained). You should also be mentally prepared. If you have been training properly, you will know how much rest you need. You should be able to relax your mind and concentrate on completing your goal.

One marathon just never seems to be enough for most people. After finishing your first marathon, you will probably say, "Never again." Your initial reaction is euphoric and you are as high as you have probably ever been. You have achieved your goal, and you think you should be able to rest on your laurels. In most cases that lasts for about one week. Then you start to remember all the training. You look at your body and know how much better you feel. You think of all the new friends you now have. They are all saying, "What marathon shall we plan for next?" and you are hooked. Now is the time to really start training. Now is the time to really improve. Now is the time to really develop that positive attitude and become committed to being a marathoner. You are ready to run for the rest of your life.

While you are training for another marathon, you can enter 5Ks and maybe become competitive. The most beautiful thing about running is that you compete within your age group. They generally give awards to the first three finishers in each age category. They generally also have an overall winner (male and female), masters winners (over forty), and grand masters (over fifty). If you are fifty, you do not have to compete against a twenty-year-old. Races are always scored in five-year age groups. Not long ago they stopped at seventy and over. More recently, most race awards go to eighty and over. I believe some time in the future age-group scoring will be raised to ninety and over. You can run or walk for the rest of your life. That is a great, happy thought.

Appendix C
A Marathon Timeline

- **Make a decision**—Choose the race you want to train for and register early.
- **Train**—Get with a group and/or a coach. It takes twenty-six weeks to train for a marathon and at least eighteen weeks for a half. (Keep in mind that you want to train so that you can run for the rest of your life.)
- **Set your biological clock**—For the week before the race, go to sleep and rise at the time you will have to do it for the race.
- **Running schedule**—Have a schedule for training that is tailored for your ability.
- **Training log**—Maintain a daily log.
- **Tapering**—Your longest, hardest run and/or walk should have been done two to three weeks before the race date. This is important to allow your body to heal. You cannot make up for training time lost.

- **Week before**—Relax, carbo load (with high fiber vegetables), have a garbage bag with a head hole prepared, check the weather report, review your race plan, take short, easy runs, and stretch.

- **Packet pick-up**—Be sure to get your packet with your scoring chip before the day of the race. There are several different types of chips, and they all come with instructions. Be sure to read them. Some chips must be returned, and others are paper that are a part of your number and can be saved or thrown away.

- **Evening preparation**—Lay out everything that you will need for the race the night before the race.

- **Men**—you probably need to protect your nipples. There are nipple protectors that are available or you can use bandaids.

- **The EXPO**—Look, see, and take samples for future use. Do not eat every sample available and have an upset stomach the next day.

- **Dry clothing**—Prepare dry clothing to take with you for when you finish.

- **Evening before**—Attach your bib number with pins to a shirt that will stay with you (front, outside). Trim your toenails. Know how to get to the starting area.

- **Race day**—Have something to eat at least one hour before race time if that is how you trained. Get to the starting area and find your corral. Hydrate. Go to the toilet if you have to. Try to do some easy stretches. You're good to go.

- **During the race**—Have a plan for what you will do during the race. This is based on your training. You should start slow for several miles and see how you feel. You should be doing negative splits, which means that you start slow and increase your pace as you get into the race. Do not try to take off fast because you will end up petering out. You should have enough energy so that you can finish with a kick. Run across that finish line with a big smile.

   Be sure that you drink and eat along the way. Do not ingest anything new that you haven't tried before. A bellyache is not what you need during a race. Talk to your neighbors, since they are probably feeling the same as you right now. This is a lot of work, but you have trained for it and know that you can finish. This is a great accomplishment, and it can be fun. Remember your mantra and yell it out if you feel like it. Everyone around you will join in and understand how you feel.

- **Protein**—Have a protein bar within thirty minutes of when you finish. Rest up and then go have a big dinner. You have earned it.

Appendix D
Injury Free Running

World class distance runners run between a 4 and 5 minute pace. Some of them have terrible form. They are lucky enough to have all the correct genes and they have probably been running almost from the time they started walking. They have eaten correctly all their lives and they have strengthened all the ligaments, tendons and muscles with a normal (for them) process while training. Most of them will run 100 to 150 miles every week. Most of them will consistently take 180 steps every minute while running. You can be envious of them but do try to copy them. Stick to the slow process of learning the correct form and increasing your distance and pace just a little at a time. Remember, as you run further and faster you should step back every four (4) weeks. Strengthen your core from your waist to the bottom of your feet. Grow gradually and learn to listen to your body.

If you have children or young relatives, try to get them interested in running and the healthy way of life. Unfortunately, we have a tendency to throw out our really good runners with the bath water. High school track and cross country coaches in many cases are not certified or qualified to train youngsters correctly. They train hard for the track season. They have a meet every week and they run competitively every week during the season. For children under the age of about sixteen (16), their skeletal frames have not fully developed. By the time they graduate from high school many of the faster runners have injuries and aches and pains and no longer can run fast. We should have more coaches that are capable of determining which students have the potential of being world class. They then can train them for the long term and not allow them to be ruined by overtraining.

If you are reading this book, you more than likely will never be world class. You may have the chance of being an elite runner, but even that depends on your early life, your genes, your competitive frame of mind, the time you have to train and improve your strength, etc. In the beginning you should just concentrate on learning the basics. Learn to run with the correct form. Learn to strengthen your entire body with particular emphasis on from the waist to the bottom of your feet. Learn to eat and hydrate properly. Get out and meet many healthy runners and make new friends. Run with other runners, but do not attempt to keep up with them, unless you are in a race. Try not to be swayed by the advice of fast runners that have no qualifications. Do some research and read. Use some common sense and take everything you hear with a grain of salt. Do not join the wild ones that go out and overtrain.

Appendix E
Running Schedules

There are all kinds of schedules available on the internet. They generally offer three (3) choices: Novice, Intermediate, Advanced

I do not know of any that suggest a track workout. I believe that a schedule should be designed for a specific individual. Schedules should start easy and can be changed for an individual that can handle a harder workout.

Train all year round. Specific training should be for 26 or 18 weeks. After your marathon take 2 or 3 weeks vacation from running. Take walks. If you have some speed, then maintain it with a track workout every week.

Howard Elakman

MARATHON TRAINING SCHEDULE
This is a sample for you to use as a base to start your own

April 2009

Monthly Planner

Done	Priority	Description	Due Date
☐		TRACK	
☐		1 MILE TIME TRIAL FIRST WEEK	

Sunday	Monday	Tuesday	Wednesday	Thursday	Friday	Saturday
Mar 2009	May 2009	*1* SAME SCHEDULE FOR APRIL AND MAY	*2* SAME SCHEDULE FOR APRIL AND MAY	*3* SAME SCHEDULE FOR APRIL AND MAY	*4* SAME SCHEDULE FOR APRIL AND MAY
5 SAME SCHEDULE FOR APRIL AND MAY	*6* SAME SCHEDULE FOR APRIL AND MAY	*7* SAME SCHEDULE FOR APRIL AND MAY	*8* SAME SCHEDULE FOR APRIL AND MAY	*9* SAME SCHEDULE FOR APRIL AND MAY	*10* SAME SCHEDULE FOR APRIL AND MAY	*11* SAME SCHEDULE FOR APRIL AND MAY
12 SAME SCHEDULE FOR APRIL AND MAY	*13* SAME SCHEDULE FOR APRIL AND MAY	*14* SAME SCHEDULE FOR APRIL AND MAY	*15* SAME SCHEDULE FOR APRIL AND MAY	*16* SAME SCHEDULE FOR APRIL AND MAY	*17* SAME SCHEDULE FOR APRIL AND MAY	*18* SAME SCHEDULE FOR APRIL AND MAY
19 SAME SCHEDULE FOR APRIL AND MAY	*20* SAME SCHEDULE FOR APRIL AND MAY	*21* SAME SCHEDULE FOR APRIL AND MAY	*22* SAME SCHEDULE FOR APRIL AND MAY	*23* SAME SCHEDULE FOR APRIL AND MAY	*24* SAME SCHEDULE FOR APRIL AND MAY	*25* SAME SCHEDULE FOR APRIL AND MAY
26 SAME SCHEDULE FOR APRIL AND MAY	*27* SAME SCHEDULE FOR APRIL AND MAY	*28* SAME SCHEDULE FOR APRIL AND MAY	*29* SAME SCHEDULE FOR APRIL AND MAY	*30* SAME SCHEDULE FOR APRIL AND MAY		

Stepping Forward

May 2009

Monthly Planner

Done	Priority	Description	Due Date
☐		TRACK	
☐		1 MILE TIME TRIAL FIRST WEEK	

Sunday	Monday	Tuesday	Wednesday	Thursday	Friday	Saturday
Apr 2009 / Jun 2009					**1** JOG on beach sand or smooth grass surface start walking and work up faster BAREFOOT	**2** REST
3 Maintenance - 10, 12 & 14 mile easy runs	**4** Easy run half the miles you do on Sunday	**5** Cross training and swimming	**6** Track workout - time trial first week - vary number of 400's and 100's reduce recovery	**7** Cross training and swimming	**8** JOG on beach sand or smooth grass surface start walking and work up faster BAREFOOT	**9** REST
10 Maintenance - 10, 12 & 14 mile easy runs	**11** Easy run half the miles you do on Sunday	**12** Cross training and swimming	**13** Track workout - time trial first week - vary number of 400's and 100's reduce recovery	**14** Cross training and swimming	**15** JOG on beach sand or smooth grass surface start walking and work up faster BAREFOOT	**16** REST
17 Maintenance - 10, 12 & 14 mile easy runs	**18** Easy run half the miles you do on Sunday	**19** Cross training and swimming	**20** Track workout - time trial first week - vary number of 400's and 100's reduce recovery	**21** Cross training and swimming	**22** JOG on beach sand or smooth grass surface start walking and work up faster BAREFOOT	**23** REST
24 Maintenance - 10, 12 & 14 mile easy runs	**25** Easy run half the miles you do on Sunday	**26** Cross training and swimming	**27** Track workout - time trial first week - vary number of 400's and 100's reduce recovery	**28** Cross training and swimming	**29** JOG on beach sand or smooth grass surface start walking and work up faster BAREFOOT	**30** REST
31 Maintenance - 10, 12 & 14 mile easy runs						

June 2009

Monthly Planner

Done	Priority	Description	Due Date
☐		TRACK	
☐		1 MILE TIME TRIAL FIRST WEEK	

Sunday	Monday	Tuesday	Wednesday	Thursday	Friday	Saturday
	1 6 MILES	**2** Strength training & stretching	**3** Track 1 mile time trial 5x400 5x100	**4** Strength training & stretching	**5** Jog barefoot on the beach or on a smooth grass surface	**6** REST
7 14 MILES	**8** 7 MILES	**9** Strength training & stretching	**10** track 6x400 6x100	**11** Strength training & stretching	**12** Jog barefoot on the beach or on a smooth grass surface	**13** REST
14 Start 18 week program training for Chicago 16 miles	**15** 9 MILES	**16** Cross train and swim	**17** track 5x800 5x100	**18** Cross train and swim	**19** Jog barefoot on the beach or on a smooth grass surface	**20** REST
21 20 miles	**22** 10 MILES	**23** Cross train and swim	**24** track 5x800 5x100	**25** Cross train and swim	**26** Jog barefoot on the beach or on a smooth grass surface	**27** REST
28 18 miles	**29** 9 MILES	**30** Cross train and swim				

Stepping Forward

July 2009

Monthly Planner

Done	Priority	Description	Due Date
☐		TRACK	
☐		1 MILE TIME TRIAL FIRST WEEK	

Sunday	Monday	Tuesday	Wednesday	Thursday	Friday	Saturday
Jun 2009 / Aug 2009			**1** TRACK - 1 MILE TIME TRIAL 5X800 5X100	**2** CROSS TRAIN / STRENGTH TRAIN	**3** 20 MINUTE TEMPO RUN - ALTERNATE W/HILLS	**4** REST
5 20 MILES	**6** 10 MILES	**7** CROSS TRAIN / STRENGTH TRAIN	**8** TRACK - start with 6x800 & 6x100 increase by one every week	**9** CROSS TRAIN / STRENGTH TRAIN	**10** 20 MINUTE TEMPO RUN - ALTERNATE W/HILLS	**11** REST
12 14 MILES	**13** 7 MILES	**14** CROSS TRAIN / STRENGTH TRAIN	**15** TRACK - start with 6x800 & 6x100 increase by one every week	**16** CROSS TRAIN / STRENGTH TRAIN	**17** 20 MINUTE TEMPO RUN - ALTERNATE W/HILLS	**18** REST
19 16 MILES	**20** 8 MILES	**21** CROSS TRAIN / STRENGTH TRAIN	**22** TRACK - start with 6x800 & 6x100 increase by one every week	**23** CROSS TRAIN / STRENGTH TRAIN	**24** 20 MINUTE TEMPO RUN - ALTERNATE W/HILLS	**25** REST
26 18 MILES	**27** 9 MILES	**28** CROSS TRAIN / STRENGTH TRAIN	**29** TRACK - start with 6x800 & 6x100 increase by one every week	**30** CROSS TRAIN / STRENGTH TRAIN	**31** 20 MINUTE TEMPO RUN - ALTERNATE W/HILLS	

Howard Elakman

August 2009

Monthly Planner

Done	Priority	Description	Due Date
☐		TRACK	
☐		1 MILE TIME TRIAL FIRST WEEK	

Sunday	Monday	Tuesday	Wednesday	Thursday	Friday	Saturday
		Jul 2009	Sep 2009			1 REST
2 20 miles	3 10 MILES	4 CROSS TRAIN STRENGTH TRAIN	5 New Event TRACK start 5x800 5x100 add 1 every week	6 CROSS TRAIN STRENGTH TRAIN	7 20 MINUTE TEMPO RUN - HILLS EVERY OTHER WEEK	8 REST
9 14 miles	10 7 MILES	11 CROSS TRAIN STRENGTH TRAIN	12 TRACK start 5x800 5x100 add 1 every week	13 CROSS TRAIN STRENGTH TRAIN	14 20 MINUTE TEMPO RUN - HILLS EVERY OTHER WEEK	15 REST
16 16 miles	17 8 MILES	18 CROSS TRAIN STRENGTH TRAIN	19 TRACK start 5x800 5x100 add 1 every week	20 CROSS TRAIN STRENGTH TRAIN	21 20 MINUTE TEMPO RUN - HILLS EVERY OTHER WEEK	22 REST
23 18 miles	24 9 MILES	25 CROSS TRAIN STRENGTH TRAIN	26 TRACK start 5x800 5x100 add 1 every week	27 CROSS TRAIN STRENGTH TRAIN	28 20 MINUTE TEMPO RUN - HILLS EVERY OTHER WEEK	29 REST
30 20 MILES race pace	31 10 MILES					

Stepping Forward

September 2009

Monthly Planner

Done	Priority	Description	Due Date
☐		TRACK	
☐		1 MILE TIME TRIAL FIRST WEEK	

Sunday	Monday	Tuesday	Wednesday	Thursday	Friday	Saturday
		1 Cross Train	*2* Track - start 9x800 - increase by one each week - 9x100 W/U & C/D	*3* Cross Train	*4* Tempo Run 20 minutes at race pace - W/U & C/D hills every other week	*5* REST
6 16 MILES - race pace	*7* 8 miles easy	*8* Cross Train	*9* Track - start 9x800 - increase by one each week - 9x100 W/U & C/D	*10* Cross Train	*11* Tempo Run 20 minutes at race pace - W/U & C/D hills every other week	*12* REST
13 18 MILES - race pace	*14* 9 miles easy	*15* Cross Train	*16* Track - start 9x800 - increase by one each week - 9x100 W/U & C/D	*17* Cross Train	*18* Tempo Run 20 minutes at race pace - W/U & C/D hills every other week	*19* REST
20 22 MILES - race pace	*21* 11 miles easy	*22* Swim	*23* Track - start 9x800 - increase by one each week - 9x100 W/U & C/D	*24* Swim	*25* Tempo Run 20 minutes at race pace - W/U & C/D hills every other week	*26* REST
27 12 MILES	*28* 6 miles easy	*29* Swim	*30* Track - 3x1mile race pace			

101

October 2009

Monthly Planner

Done	Priority	Description	Due Date
☐		TRACK	
☐		1 MILE TIME TRIAL FIRST WEEK	

Sunday	Monday	Tuesday	Wednesday	Thursday	Friday	Saturday
Sep 2009		Nov 2009		1 SWIM	2 Some easy hill runs	3 REST
4 8 MILES	5 5 MILES	6 4 MILES	7 3 MILES 1 mile at race pace	8 2 MILES	9 2 MILES	10 REST
11 Chicago Marathon	12	13	14	15	16	17
18	19	20	21	22	23	24
25	26	27	28	29	30	31

Stepping Forward

HALF MARATHON SCHEDULE

May 2009

Monthly Planner

Done	Priority	Description	Due Date

Sunday	Monday	Tuesday	Wednesday	Thursday	Friday	Saturday
Apr 2009 S M T W T F S 1 2 3 4 5 6 7 8 9 10 11 12 13 14 15 16 17 18 19 20 21 22 23 24 25 26 27 28 29 30	*Jun 2009* S M T W T F S 1 2 3 4 5 6 7 8 9 10 11 12 13 14 15 16 17 18 19 20 21 22 23 24 25 26 27 28 29 30				**1** TEMPO RUN - run fast - start with 1 or 2 minutes and add 1 minute each week	**2** REST
3 6 MILES W/ fartlik every 2 miles stretch when finished	**4** 3 miles easy - practise your running form - RUN WITH YOUR HANDS	**5** CROSS TRAIN	**6** TRACK - start w/ 2x400 w/ 200 recovery add 1 more each week - 2x100 fast walk back	**7** CROSS TRAIN	**8** TEMPO RUN - run fast - start with 1 or 2 minutes and add 1 minute each week	**9** REST Run For The Roses 5K Markham Park
10 6 MILES W/ fartlik every 2 miles stretch when finished	**11** 3 miles easy - practise your running form - RUN WITH YOUR HANDS	**12** CROSS TRAIN	**13** TRACK - start w/ 2x400 w/ 200 recovery add 1 more each week - 2x100 fast walk back	**14** CROSS TRAIN	**15** TEMPO RUN - run fast - start with 1 or 2 minutes and add 1 minute each week	**16** REST
17 6 MILES W/ fartlik every 2 miles stretch when finished	**18** 3 miles easy - practise your running form - RUN WITH YOUR HANDS	**19** CROSS TRAIN	**20** TRACK - start w/ 2x400 w/ 200 recovery add 1 more each week - 2x100 fast walk back	**21** CROSS TRAIN	**22** TEMPO RUN - run fast - start with 1 or 2 minutes and add 1 minute each week	**23** REST
24 6 MILES W/ fartlik every 2 miles stretch when finished	**25** 3 miles easy - practise your running form - RUN WITH YOUR HANDS	**26** CROSS TRAIN	**27** TRACK - start w/ 2x400 w/ 200 recovery add 1 more each week - 2x100 fast walk back	**28** CROSS TRAIN	**29** TEMPO RUN - run fast - start with 1 or 2 minutes and add 1 minute each week	**30** REST
31 6 MILES W/ fartlik every 2 miles stretch when finished						

June 2009

Monthly Planner

Done	Priority	Description	Due Date

Sunday	Monday	Tuesday	Wednesday	Thursday	Friday	Saturday
	1 3 TO 4 MILES EASY	2 CROSS TRAIN	3 TRACK - start w/ 2x400 and add 1 each week 200 recovery 2x100 walk back +1 each week	4 CROSS TRAIN	5 Tempo Run - fairly fast for 2 or 3 minutes - always warm up before & cool down after	6 REST
7 8 miles w/ fartlik every 2 miles	8 3 TO 4 MILES EASY	9 CROSS TRAIN	10 TRACK - start w/ 2x400 and add 1 each week 200 recovery 2x100 walk back +1 each week	11 CROSS TRAIN	12 HILLS - find a place where you can run up a hill on grass run hard 2 or 3 times walk down	13 REST
14 6 miles easy w/ fartlik every 2 miles	15 3 TO 4 MILES EASY	16 CROSS TRAIN	17 TRACK - start w/ 2x400 and add 1 each week 200 recovery 2x100 walk back +1 each week	18 CROSS TRAIN	19 Tempo Run - fairly fast for 2 or 3 minutes - always warm up before & cool down after	20 REST
21 8 miles w/ fartlik every 2 miles	22 3 TO 4 MILES EASY	23 CROSS TRAIN	24 TRACK - start w/ 2x400 and add 1 each week 200 recovery 2x100 walk back +1 each week	25 CROSS TRAIN	26 HILLS - find a place where you can run up a hill on grass run hard 2 or 3 times walk down	27 Freedom 5K Quiet Waters Park REST
28 6 miles easy w/ fartlik every 2 miles	29 3 TO 4 MILES EASY	30 CROSS TRAIN				

Stepping Forward

July 2009

Monthly Planner

Done	Priority	Description	Due Date

Sunday	Monday	Tuesday	Wednesday	Thursday	Friday	Saturday
Jun 2009 / Aug 2009			**1** TRACK - 2x400 w/ 200 recovery 1x800 w/ 400 recovery	**2** CROSS TRAIN	**3** Tempo Run - 2 to 5 minutes at your 10K pace	**4** REST
5 8 miles easy w/ fartlik every mile	**6** 4 MILES EASY	**7** CROSS TRAIN	**8** TRACK - 3x400 w/ 200 recovery 1x800 4/ 400 recovery 2x100 walk back	**9** CROSS TRAIN	**10** Hills - Find a grass hill & run up hard 4 to 5 times walk down	**11** REST
12 10 miles easy w/ fartlik every mile	**13** 5 MILES EASY	**14** CROSS TRAIN	**15** TRACK - 3x400 w/ 200 recovery 1x800 4/ 400 recovery 2x100 walk back	**16** CROSS TRAIN	**17** Tempo Run - 2 to 5 minutes at your 10K pace	**18** Dreher Park 5K West Palm Beach REST
19 6 miles easy w/fartlik every mile	**20** 3 MILES EASY	**21** CROSS TRAIN	**22** TRACK - 4x400 w/ 200 recovery 1x800 w/ 400 recovery 3x100 walk back	**23** CROSS TRAIN	**24** Hills - Find a grass hill & run up hard 4 to 5 times walk down	**25** REST
26 8 miles easy w/fartlik every mile	**27** 4 MILES EASY	**28** CROSS TRAIN	**29** TRACK - 4x400 w/ 200 recovery 1x800 w/ 400 recovery 3x100 walk back	**30** CROSS TRAIN	**31** Tempo Run - 2 to 5 minutes at your 10K pace	

Howard Elakman

August 2009

Monthly Planner

Done	Priority	Description	Due Date

Sunday	Monday	Tuesday	Wednesday	Thursday	Friday	Saturday
		Jul 2009	Sep 2009			**1** REST
2 10 miles slow w/ fartlik each mile	**3** 5 MILES EASY	**4** CROSS TRAIN	**5** TRACK - start this month w/ 3x800 +1 ea. week - 3x100 +1 each week	**6** CROSS TRAIN	**7** tempo run - 5 to 10 minutes	**8** ING Miami Marathon Kick Off 5K Hugh Taylor Birch Park REST
9 12 miles slow w/ fartlik each mile	**10** 6 MILES EASY	**11** CROSS TRAIN	**12** TRACK - start this month w/ 3x800 +1 ea. week - 3x100 +1 each week	**13** CROSS TRAIN	**14** hill workout - 4 or 5 times up and walk down	**15** REST
16 6 miles w/ fartlik each mile	**17** 3 MILES EASY	**18** CROSS TRAIN	**19** TRACK - start this month w/ 3x800 +1 ea. week - 3x100 +1 each week	**20** CROSS TRAIN	**21** tempo run - 5 to 10 minutes	**22** REST
23 8 miles w/ fartlik each mile	**24** 4 MILES EASY	**25** CROSS TRAIN	**26** TRACK - start this month w/ 3x800 +1 ea. week - 3x100 +1 each week	**27** CROSS TRAIN	**28** hill workout - 4 or 5 times up and walk down	**29** REST
30 10 MILES - slow with fartlik each mile	**31** 5 MILES EASY					

Stepping Forward

September 2009

Monthly Planner

Done	Priority	Description	Due Date

Sunday	Monday	Tuesday	Wednesday	Thursday	Friday	Saturday
		1 CROSS TRAIN	2 TRACK - start with 5x800 w 400 or less recovery - +1 each week 5x100 +1 ea.week	3 CROSS TRAIN	4 Tempo Run - build up to 20 minutes slowly each week - alternate with hills	5 REST
6 12 miles - a bit slower than race pace	7 6 miles easy	8 CROSS TRAIN	9 TRACK - start with 5x800 w 400 or less recovery - +1 each week 5x100 +1 ea.week	10 CROSS TRAIN	11 Tempo Run - build up to 20 minutes slowly each week - alternate with hills	12 Fall Fling 5K Tradewinds Park REST
13 6 miles - try to maintain race pace	14 3 miles easy	15 CROSS TRAIN	16 TRACK - start with 5x800 w 400 or less recovery - +1 each week 5x100 +1 ea.week	17 CROSS TRAIN	18 Tempo Run - build up to 20 minutes slowly each week - alternate with hills	19 REST
20 8 miles - try to maintain race pace	21 4 miles easy	22 CROSS TRAIN	23 TRACK - start with 5x800 w 400 or less recovery - +1 each week 5x100 +1 ea.week	24 CROSS TRAIN	25 Tempo Run - build up to 20 minutes slowly each week - alternate with hills	26 REST
27 10 MILES try to maintain race pace	28 5 miles easy	29 CROSS TRAIN	30 TRACK - start with 5x800 w 400 or less recovery - +1 each week 5x100 +1 ea.week			

Howard Elakman

October 2009

Monthly Planner

Done	Priority	Description	Due Date

Sunday	Monday	Tuesday	Wednesday	Thursday	Friday	Saturday
Sep 2009 / Nov 2009				**1** CROSS TRAIN	**2** Tempo Run for 20 minutes - alternate each week with hill workout	**3** REST
4 12 miles at 30 seconds slower than race pace	**5** 6 miles 1 minute slower than race pace	**6** CROSS TRAIN	**7** TRACK - start this month with 7x800 w/ 400 or less recovery-add 1 each week-7x100	**8** CROSS TRAIN	**9** Tempo Run for 20 minutes - alternate each week with hill workout	**10** REST
11 6 miles race pace	**12** 3 miles 1 min. slower than race pace	**13** CROSS TRAIN	**14** TRACK - start this month with 7x800 w/ 400 or less recovery-add 1 each week-7x100	**15** CROSS TRAIN	**16** Tempo Run for 20 minutes - alternate each week with hill workout	**17** REST
18 8 miles race pace	**19** 4 miles slower than race pace	**20** CROSS TRAIN	**21** TRACK - start this month with 7x800 w/ 400 or less recovery-add 1 each week-7x100	**22** CROSS TRAIN	**23** Tempo Run for 20 minutes - alternate each week with hill workout	**24** REST
25 10 miles race pace	**26** 5 miles - 1 min. slower than race pace	**27** CROSS TRAIN	**28** TRACK - start this month with 7x800 w/ 400 or less recovery-add 1 each week-7x100	**29** CROSS TRAIN	**30** Tempo Run for 20 minutes - alternate each week with hill workout	**31** REST Spooktacular 5K TY Park, Hollywood

Stepping Forward

November 2009

Monthly Planner

Done	Priority	Description	Due Date

Sunday	Monday	Tuesday	Wednesday	Thursday	Friday	Saturday
1 12 miles at race pace	**2** Start tapering - easy 6 miles	**3** easy 3 miles	**4** Run a few half mile repeats to wake up your fast twitch muscles	**5** Walk 3 miles on a soft surface barefoot	**6** Tempo run for 15 minutes - warm & cool down	**7** Go for a nice stroll of 3 or 4 miles
8 8 miles easy	**9** easy 4 miles	**10** easy 3 miles	**11** 4 miles easy	**12** Walk 3 miles on a soft surface barefoot	**13** easy 3 miles	**14** Go for a nice stroll of 3 or 4 miles
15 13.1 Marathon Ft. Lauderdale	**16** Walk a bit and rest	**17** Walk a bit and rest	**18** Walk a bit and rest	**19** Walk a bit and rest	**20** Walk a bit and rest	**21** Walk a bit and rest
22 Walk a bit and rest	**23** Walk a bit and rest	**24** Walk a bit and rest	**25** Walk a bit and rest	**26** Walk a bit and rest	**27** Walk a bit and rest	**28** Walk a bit and rest
29	**30**					

References

Benson, R. *The Runner's Coach.* Tallahassee: Cedarwinds, 1998.

———. *Coach Benson's "Secret" Workouts.* New York: Beaufort Books, 2003.

Benson, T., and I. Ray. *Run with the Best.* Mountain View: Tafnews Press, 2001.

Daniels, J. *Daniels' Running Formula.* Champaign: Human Kinetics Publishers, 2005.

Drum, T. *'Fraid Nots.* Pompano Beach: Tom Drum Inc, 1996.

Floyd, P. A., and J. Parke. *Walk, Jog, Run, for Wellness Everyone.* Winston-Salem: Hunter Textbooks, 1996.

Gold, R. *Thai Massage: A Traditional Medical Technique.* Philadelphia: Mosby, 2001.

Mattes, A. *Specific Stretching for Everyone.* Sarasota; Aaron L. Mattes, 2000.

Mercati, M. *Thai Massage Manual: Natural Therapy for Flexibility, Relaxation, and Energy Balance.* New York: Sterling Publishing, 2005.

Shaw, B. *Beth Shaw's YogaFit.* Champaign: Human Kinetics Publishers, 2008.

Ungaro, A. *Pilates: Body in Motion.* London: Dorling Kindersley Limited, 2002.

Walker, Brad. *The Stretching Handbook.* Australia: The Stretching Institute.

Willett, W.C. *Eat, Drink, and Be Healthy.* New York: Free Press, 2001.

Yessis, M. *Explosive Running.* Columbus: McGraw-Hill, 2000.

LaVergne, TN USA
28 March 2010
177369LV00002B/17/P